Genetic Perspectives in
Thyroid Cancer

Genetic Perspectives in Thyroid Cancer

Editor

Susana Nunes Silva

MDPI • Basel • Beijing • Wuhan • Barcelona • Belgrade • Manchester • Tokyo • Cluj • Tianjin

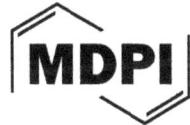

Editor
Susana Nunes Silva
Centre for Toxicogenomics and
Human Health, Genetics,
Oncology and Human Toxicology,
NOVA Medical School—Faculdade de Ciências Médicas,
Universidade Nova de Lisboa
Portugal

Editorial Office
MDPI
St. Alban-Anlage 66
4052 Basel, Switzerland

This is a reprint of articles from the Special Issue published online in the open access journal *Genes* (ISSN 2073-4425) (available at: https://www.mdpi.com/journal/genes/special_issues/Genetic_Thyroid_Cancer).

For citation purposes, cite each article independently as indicated on the article page online and as indicated below:

LastName, A.A.; LastName, B.B.; LastName, C.C. Article Title. *Journal Name* **Year**, *Volume Number*, Page Range.

ISBN 978-3-0365-0544-2 (Hbk)
ISBN 978-3-0365-0545-9 (PDF)

© 2021 by the authors. Articles in this book are Open Access and distributed under the Creative Commons Attribution (CC BY) license, which allows users to download, copy and build upon published articles, as long as the author and publisher are properly credited, which ensures maximum dissemination and a wider impact of our publications.

The book as a whole is distributed by MDPI under the terms and conditions of the Creative Commons license CC BY-NC-ND.

Contents

About the Editor vii

Susana Nunes Silva
Special Issue: Genetic Perspectives in Thyroid Cancer
Reprinted from: *Genes* **2021**, *12*, 126, doi:10.3390/genes12020126 1

Paul J. Davis, Hung-Yun Lin, Aleck Hercbergs and Shaker A. Mousa
Actions of L-thyroxine (T4) and Tetraiodothyroacetic Acid (Tetrac) on Gene Expression in Thyroid Cancer Cells
Reprinted from: *Genes* **2020**, *11*, 755, doi:10.3390/genes11070755 3

Leonardo P. Stuchi, Márcia Maria U. Castanhole-Nunes, Nathália Maniezzo-Stuchi, Patrícia M. Biselli-Chicote, Tiago Henrique, João Armando Padovani Neto, Dalisio de-Santi Neto, Ana Paula Girol, Erika C. Pavarino and Eny Maria Goloni-Bertollo
VEGFA and *NFE2L2* Gene Expression and Regulation by MicroRNAs in Thyroid Papillary Cancer and Colloid Goiter
Reprinted from: *Genes* **2020**, *11*, 954, doi:10.3390/genes11090954 13

Dumitru A. Iacobas
Biomarkers, Master Regulators and Genomic Fabric Remodeling in a Case of Papillary Thyroid Carcinoma
Reprinted from: *Genes* **2020**, *11*, 1030, doi:10.3390/genes11091030 27

Soo-Hwan Byun, Chanyang Min, Hyo-Geun Choi and Seok-Jin Hong
Association between Family Histories of Thyroid Cancer and Thyroid Cancer Incidence: A Cross-Sectional Study Using the Korean Genome and Epidemiology Study Data
Reprinted from: *Genes* **2020**, *11*, 1039, doi:10.3390/genes11091039 49

Luís S. Santos, Octávia M. Gil, Susana N. Silva, Bruno C. Gomes, Teresa C. Ferreira, Edward Limbert and José Rueff
Micronuclei Formation upon Radioiodine Therapy for Well-Differentiated Thyroid Cancer: The Influence of DNA Repair Genes Variants
Reprinted from: *Genes* **2020**, *11*, 1083, doi:10.3390/genes11091083 61

Fabíola Yukiko Miasaki, Cesar Seigi Fuziwara, Gisah Amaral de Carvalho and Edna Teruko Kimura
Genetic Mutations and Variants in the Susceptibility of Familial Non-Medullary Thyroid Cancer
Reprinted from: *Genes* **2020**, *11*, 1364, doi:10.3390/genes11111364 87

About the Editor

Susana Nunes Silva was born in Lisbon in 1978. In 2002, she received her 5-year graduation degree in Biotechnology Engineering, and in 2010, her PhD in Life Sciences Field Genetics from Faculdade Ciências Médicas—Universidade Nova de Lisboa (FCM—UNL). During the PhD, she collaborated as an assistant in genetic pratical classes to medical students, lecturing since her master's and doctoral courses. In September 2015, she became an Invited Assistant Teacher in Integrated Master Degree in Medicine Lecturing Genetics in FCM. She has been involved in the training and supervision of several graduation, master's and PhD students. In research, the main field of interest has been oncobiology and toxicology (breast and thyroid cancer) as a researcher in DNA Damage and Repair Group from Centre for Toxicogenomics and Human Health from NOVA Medical School, Universidade Nova e Lisboa.

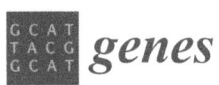

Editorial

Special Issue: Genetic Perspectives in Thyroid Cancer

Susana Nunes Silva

Centre for Toxicogenomics and Human Health (ToxOmics), Genetics, Oncology and Human Toxicology, NOVA Medical School, Faculdade de Ciências Médicas, Universidade Nova de Lisboa, 1169-056 Lisboa, Portugal; snsilva@nms.unl.pt

Received: 30 December 2020; Accepted: 15 January 2021; Published: 20 January 2021

Thyroid cancer is not just a common type of cancer, it is the most frequently diagnosed endocrine malignancy worldwide. The aetiology of thyroid cancer is essentially multifactorial and radiation is the best documented risk factor related to the disease. However, many questions are still open and seeking clarification, especially regarding the genetic aspects of this pathology, with clear implications not only on a scientific basis of the disease, but foremost in clinical oncology.

Thyroid gland tumours are a heterogeneous group of neoplasms that may arise from virtually any of the different cell types that are present in the thyroid gland. Although the malignant tumours are most frequently identified in thyroid follicular cells, it is clear that the molecular-genetic characterization is crucial and should be further explored to emphasize differences in tumour biological behaviours, aggressiveness, and disease prognostics. Papillary and follicular thyroid carcinomas (PTC and FTC, respectively) represent 85–90% and 5–10% of thyroid cancer cases, respectively, arising from thyroid follicular cells. These tumour histotypes retain their morphologic features and are often referred to as differentiated thyroid carcinoma (DTC). However, the aetiology of DTC is still unknown.

Considerable progress has been made in the understanding of thyroid carcinogenesis, in part based on retrospective and prospective studies published worldwide in recent decades, but also in the development of high-throughput approaches and the availability of improved diagnostic methodologies that lead to early diagnosis. In fact, over the last few decades, the research in thyroid cancer has highlighted the mutational landscape leading to better understanding of the molecular pathogenesis of DTC.

The hallmarks of cancer have been identified with several potential targets involved in gene expression deregulation, leading to the promotion of genetic instability and cancer development. The identification of genetic variants related to thyroid cancer has been a long way, though it is crucial to identify possible potential biomarkers of susceptibility. Some genetic variants have been identified in specific subtypes, which are related to the increased risk to develop this malignancy, such as the *BRAF* V600E mutation in PTC patients with a more aggressive phenotype if *TERT* promoter mutation coexists [1]. However, mutations in *RET* and *RAS* genes have also been identified as biomarkers in thyroid cancer patients.

Alongside with genetic variants, epigenetic events and alterations in the expression of microRNAs (miRNAs) [2] and long noncoding RNAs (lncRNA) may also, through modulation of gene expression [3], drive the aberrant activation of oncogenic signalling pathways and the downregulation of thyroid-specific genes, thus contributing to the development, progression, and dedifferentiation of thyroid cancer [4].

Connected to this, the genetic instability inflicted in this malignancy, involving genetic and epigenetic alterations, might also compromise the treatment response. The standard treatment for thyroid cancer patients consists of surgical resection accompanied by post-thyroidectomy radioiodine (RAI) adjuvant therapy. The radioiodine therapy relies on the ability of 131I to be preferentially taken up in normal or neoplastic thyroid follicular cells. Its accumulation induces high DNA damage, which leads to cytotoxicity. However, the ionizing radiation does not only affect tumour cells, but the lesions may also impair normal cells. The most common lesions induced by radiation are double-strand breaks (DSBs), which are processed by enzymes involved in DNA repair pathways. The presence of genetic variants in these enzymes might impair the repair efficiency but also could influence the cytotoxic potential of RAI therapy, hence its efficacy in DTC treatment [5]. The development of induced DNA damage approaches can help in the evaluation of the efficacy of therapeutics as it has been shown to be an important tool for establishing biomarkers of susceptibility.

Although the most frequent variants identified in thyroid cancer contribute to sporadic disease, about 5 to 15% of all diagnosed cases are familial (first degree relatives) in nonmedullary thyroid cancer (NMTC), increasing to 25% in medullary thyroid cancer (MTC) cases. This adds to the clear existence of genetic predisposition factors related to this pathology [6]. Advances in molecular genetics and several candidate gene studies developed worldwide have linked the occurrence of this malignancy to some hereditary syndromes, some of which are related to germline mutations in *RET* genes.

Although thyroid cancer is not considered a common malignancy, with a 98% relative survival rate, this does not undermine the need to fully understand the mechanisms of disease in all of its aspects using all available tools from epidemiology approaches—genetic, epigenetic, regulation, therapeutic response, and resistance [7].

This collection aims to show how much has been achieved and what remains to be done with regard to thyroid cancer. Above all, bringing together researchers and clinicians is the key to better understand this heterogeneous disease.

Funding: This research received no external funding.

Conflicts of Interest: The author declares no conflict of interest.

References

1. Luzon-Toro, B.; Fernandez, R.M.; Villalba-Benito, L.; Torroglosa, A.; Antinolo, G.; Borrego, S. Influencers on Thyroid Cancer Onset: Molecular Genetic Basis. *Genes* **2019**, *10*, 913. [CrossRef] [PubMed]
2. Stuchi, L.P.; Castanhole-Nunes, M.M.U.; Maniezzo-Stuchi, N.; Biselli-Chicote, P.M.; Henrique, T.; Padovani Neto, J.A.; de-Santi Neto, D.; Girol, A.P.; Pavarino, E.C.; Goloni-Bertollo, E.M. VEGFA and NFE2L2 Gene Expression and Regulation by MicroRNAs in Thyroid Papillary Cancer and Colloid Goiter. *Genes* **2020**, *11*, 954. [CrossRef] [PubMed]
3. Davis, P.J.; Lin, H.Y.; Hercbergs, A.; Mousa, S.A. Actions of L-thyroxine (T4) and Tetraiodothyroacetic Acid (Tetrac) on Gene Expression in Thyroid Cancer Cells. *Genes* **2020**, *11*, 755. [CrossRef] [PubMed]
4. Iacobas, D.A. Biomarkers, Master Regulators and Genomic Fabric Remodeling in a Case of Papillary Thyroid Carcinoma. *Genes* **2020**, *11*, 1030. [CrossRef] [PubMed]
5. Santos, L.S.; Monteiro-Gil, O.; Silva, S.N.; Gomes, B.C.; Ferreira, T.C.; Limbert, E.; Rueff, J. Micronuclei Formation upon Radioiodine Therapy for Well-Differentiated Thyroid Cancer: The Influence of DNA Repair Genes Variants. *Genes* **2020**, *11*, 1083. [CrossRef] [PubMed]
6. Miasaki, F.Y.; Fuziwara, C.S.; Carvalho, G.A.; Kimura, E.T. Genetic Mutations and Variants in the Susceptibility of Familial Non-Medullary Thyroid Cancer. *Genes* **2020**, *11*, 1364. [CrossRef] [PubMed]
7. Byun, S.H.; Min, C.; Choi, H.G.; Hong, S.J. Association between Family Histories of Thyroid Cancer and Thyroid Cancer Incidence: A Cross-Sectional Study Using the Korean Genome and Epidemiology Study Data. *Genes* **2020**, *11*, 1039. [CrossRef] [PubMed]

Publisher's Note: MDPI stays neutral with regard to jurisdictional claims in published maps and institutional affiliations.

© 2021 by the author. Licensee MDPI, Basel, Switzerland. This article is an open access article distributed under the terms and conditions of the Creative Commons Attribution (CC BY) license (http://creativecommons.org/licenses/by/4.0/).

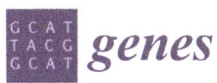

Review

Actions of L-thyroxine (T4) and Tetraiodothyroacetic Acid (Tetrac) on Gene Expression in Thyroid Cancer Cells

Paul J. Davis [1,2,*], Hung-Yun Lin [3,4,5], Aleck Hercbergs [6] and Shaker A. Mousa [2]

1. Department of Medicine, Albany Medical College, Albany, NY 12208, USA
2. Pharmaceutical Research Institute, Albany College of Pharmacy and Health Sciences, Rensselaer, NY 12144, USA; shaker.mousa@acphs.edu
3. Ph.D. Program for Cancer Molecular Biology and Drug Discovery, College of Medical Science and Technology, Taipei Medical University, Taipei 11031, Taiwan; linhy@tmu.edu.tw
4. Cancer Center, Wan Fang Hospital, Taipei Medical University, Taipei 11031, Taiwan
5. Traditional Herbal Medicine Research Center of Taipei Medical University Hospital, Taipei Medical University, Taipei 11031, Taiwan
6. Department of Radiation Oncology, The Cleveland Clinic, Cleveland, OH 44195, USA; hercbergs@gmail.com
* Correspondence: pdavis.ordwayst@gmail.com

Received: 10 June 2020; Accepted: 1 July 2020; Published: 7 July 2020

Abstract: The clinical behavior of thyroid cancers is seen to reflect inherent transcriptional activities of mutated genes and trophic effects on tumors of circulating pituitary thyrotropin (TSH). The thyroid hormone, L-thyroxine (T4), has been shown to stimulate proliferation of a large number of different forms of cancer. This activity of T4 is mediated by a cell surface receptor on the extracellular domain of integrin $\alpha v \beta 3$. In this brief review, we describe what is known about T4 as a circulating trophic factor for differentiated (papillary and follicular) thyroid cancers. Given T4's cancer-stimulating activity in differentiated thyroid cancers, it was not surprising to find that genomic actions of T4 were anti-apoptotic. Transduction of the T4-generated signal at the integrin primarily involved mitogen-activated protein kinase (MAPK). In thyroid C cell-origin medullary carcinoma of the thyroid (MTC), effects of thyroid hormone analogues, such as tetraiodothyroacetic acid (tetrac), include pro-angiogenic and apoptosis-linked genes. Tetrac is an inhibitor of the actions of T4 at $\alpha v \beta 3$, and it is assumed, but not yet proved, that the anti-angiogenic and pro-apoptotic actions of tetrac in MTC cells are matched by T4 effects that are pro-angiogenic and anti-apoptotic. We also note that papillary thyroid carcinoma cells may express the leptin receptor, and circulating leptin from adipocytes may stimulate tumor cell proliferation. Transcription was stimulated by leptin in anaplastic, papillary, and follicular carcinomas of genes involved in invasion, such as matrix metalloproteinases (MMPs). In summary, thyroid hormone analogues may act at their receptor on integrin $\alpha v \beta 3$ in a variety of types of thyroid cancer to modulate transcription of genes relevant to tumor invasiveness, apoptosis, and angiogenesis. These effects are independent of TSH.

Keywords: apoptosis; angiogenesis; integrin $\alpha v \beta 3$; L-thyroxine (T4); thyroid cancer; tetraiodothyroacetic acid (tetrac)

1. Introduction

The clinical behavior of thyroid gland cancers is seen to reflect gene mutation and/or epigenetic changes [1,2], and effects of circulating or local trophic factors [3,4]. Circulating trophic factors include target tissue-specific thyrotropin (TSH) secreted by the pituitary gland and adipose tissue-source leptin, which enhances growth of a variety of tumors, including those of the thyroid gland [5]. In the clinical management of differentiated thyroid cancers, host pituitary TSH secretion is suppressed with exogenous L-thyroxine (T4) in conjunction with tumor surgery and radioablation of the cancers.

Discovery of a cell surface thyroid hormone analogue receptor on plasma membrane integrin αvβ3 has provided additional information about the biological activity of T4. T4 has been viewed primarily as a source of 3,3′,5-triiodo-L-thyronine (T3), the principally active form of the hormone at nuclear thyroid hormone receptors (TRs) [6,7]. At physiological concentrations, however, T4 is the primary ligand of the cell surface iodothyronine receptor on the plasma membrane [8]. The integrin is generously expressed by cancer cells and rapidly dividing endothelial cells [6] and at this site, T4 promotes proliferation of tumor cells and supports angiogenesis [8]. T4 may also be a factor that contributes to metastasis of cancer cells [9].

Reverse T3 (3,3′,5′-triiodo-L-thyronine, rT3) has also been thought to have little bioactivity but is known to affect the state of actin in cells [10] and, recently, to stimulate proliferation of cancer cells [11]. In contrast to T4 and to rT3, tetraiodothyroacetic acid (tetrac), a derivative of T4, has anti-proliferative and anti-angiogenic properties at αvβ3 [6,8,12]. Prior to recognition of anti-tumor activity of tetrac at the cell surface integrin, tetrac was seen to have low-grade T3-like activity at the nuclear receptors [6].

Against this background, we examine in the present review the actions of T4 and tetrac, and chemical derivatives of tetrac on the biology of human thyroid cancer cells, including expression of a number of genes relevant to proliferation, apoptosis, and angiogenesis. These actions of T4 and tetrac are initiated at the hormone receptor on integrin αvβ3 (Figure 1). The signals generated at the integrin by thyroid hormone analogues involve early transduction within the cell primarily by mitogen-activated protein kinase (MAPK) [6,8].

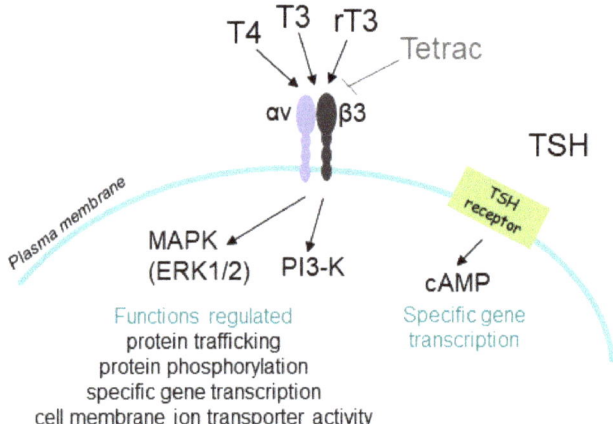

Figure 1. Cancer-relevant actions of thyroid hormones and pituitary thyrotropin (TSH) at thyroid carcinoma cells. Plasma membrane integrin αvβ3 contains a cell surface receptor for thyroid hormones and is overexpressed by cancer cells. T4 is the principal ligand for this receptor and the T4 signal is transduced by mitogen-activated protein kinase (MAPK/ERK1/2) or phosphatidylinositol 3-kinase (PI3-K) into cancer-linked gene transcription. A deaminated analogue of T4, tetrac, blocks actions of T4 at the integrin and is under development as an anticancer agent. At physiological concentrations, T3 is not active at the integrin, but reverse T3 (rT3) has cancer cell-stimulating activity at this plasma membrane receptor. T3 is the principal ligand of nuclear thyroid hormone receptors (TRs) in normal cells; TRs are not shown in the figure. Pituitary TSH acts at a specific cAMP-generating receptor on the plasma membrane of thyroid cancer cells. TRs and the TSH receptor are not structurally related to the T4 binding site on αvβ3. 2. T4 Actions at the Integrin αvβ3 in Papillary and Follicular Thyroid Carcinoma Cells.

2. T4 Actions at the Integrin αvβ3 in Papillary and Follicular Thyroid Carcinoma Cells

The physiological loops that connect the components of the normal hypothalamic-pituitary-thyroid gland axis have been assumed to be intact when the axis is disrupted by thyroid cancer [3,6,13–15]. In differentiated thyroid cancers, the tumor cells are usually TSH-responsive in terms of proliferation and pharmacologic administration of thyroid hormone—as T4, serving as a source of T3 at the level of nuclear TRs in the pituitary—and can take advantage of the thyro-pituitary feedback loop and suppress endogenous thyrotropin. The reduction of circulating TSH frequently contributes to arrest of the thyroid cancer. The amounts of exogenous T4 that are required to fully suppress host TSH via generated T3 are, by the nature of the definition of the feedback loop, supraphysiologic. The thyroid hormone receptors involved are exclusively nuclear TRs.

Lin et al. [16] showed in 2007 that differentiated papillary and follicular human thyroid carcinoma cells in vitro proliferated in response to physiological levels of T4. The index of cell division was expression of proliferating cell nuclear antigen (PCNA) (see Figure 2). The proliferative effect of T4 was inhibited by tetrac that, as noted above, blocks actions of T4 that are initiated at integrin αvβ3. An Arg-Gly-Asp (RGD) peptide that acts on a number of integrins and has a receptor close to the T4 receptor on αvβ3, also blocked the action of T4 on thyroid cancer cells, but a control Arg-Gly-Glu (RGE) peptide did not affect the action of T4. This report, thus, documented a local and primary effect of the principal hormonal product of the thyroid gland on thyroid gland cancer cells. TSH was not involved. The cell lines in this work had been well-studied by other endocrine laboratories and were the subjects of more than 20 publications.

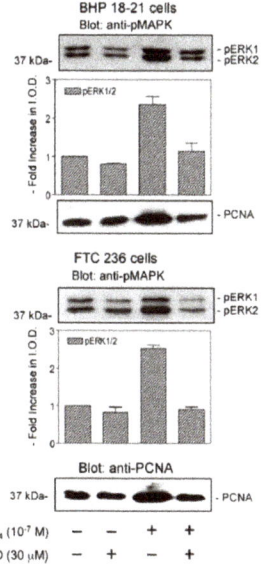

Figure 2. Proliferative activity of T4 in vitro on differentiated human papillary (BHP 18-21; upper panel) and follicular (FTC 236: lower panel) thyroid carcinoma cells. Proliferation was measured by immunoblotting of proliferative cell nuclear antigen (PCNA) from cultured cells. The 2.5-fold increase in PCNA in both cell lines was achieved with 10^{-7} M total T4 concentration (10^{-10} M free T4 in medium) [17]. The proliferative effect of the hormone required activation of ERK1/2 (MAPK). Inhibition of activation of ERK1/2 with PD98059 (PD) prevented enhancement of proliferation in both cell lines. T4 activates MAPK via the thyroid hormone analogue receptor on the extracellular domain of plasma membrane integrin αvβ3 [8,17]. Reprinted with permission from Elsevier from Lin et al. [16]. ERK1/2, extracellular signal-regulated kinases 1 and 2; MAPK, mitogen-activated protein kinase.

Another feature of the Lin et al. study was to define molecular components of the mechanism, downstream of its receptor on the integrin [8,16,17] by which T4 stimulated cell proliferation. That activation of MAPK was essential to the induction of proliferation was shown with the use of pharmacologic inhibitor of MAPK [18] (Figure 2), which eliminated the stimulatory T4 action on PCNA. The requirement for MAPK participation in T4's action on proliferation has been shown in a number of cancer cells [19–25]. Only at supraphysiologic concentrations was T3 effective as a proliferative factor [16] and this is a feature of cancer cell responses that are mediated by the receptor for thyroid hormone on integrin $\alpha v\beta 3$ [17].

To define the specific genes whose transcription is affected by T4, Lin and co-workers [16] studied the effects of T4 on pharmacologically induced apoptosis in papillary and follicular thyroid cancer cells. The stilbene, resveratrol, induces apoptosis in differentiated thyroid cancer cells by a complex molecular mechanism that involves *p21*, *c-Jun*, and *c-Fos* expression [26]. As shown in Figure 3, resveratrol activated pro-apoptotic p53 and increased cancer cell expression of *p21*, *c-Fos*, and *c-Jun* genes. Addition of T4 to the cells cultured with resveratrol prevented p53 activation and apoptosis and also blocked induction of expression of *p21*, *c-Jun*, and *c-Fos*. Thus, T4 has anti-apoptotic activity in thyroid cancer cells by multiple mechanisms, including expression of multiple genes and reversing activation of p53. It is also important to note that tetrac inhibited resveratrol-induced apoptosis, as shown in nucleosome ELISA studies [16]. The anti-apoptosis effects of T4 in these studies, like those on cell proliferation, are initiated at the cell surface thyroid hormone receptor on integrin $\alpha v\beta 3$.

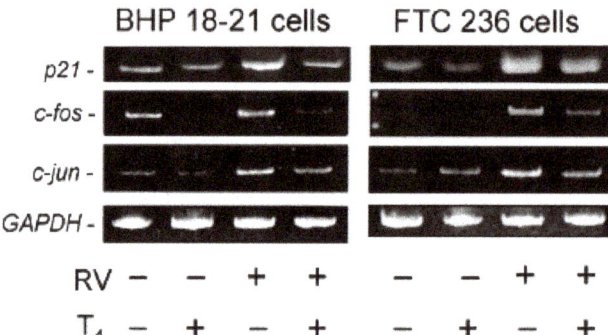

Figure 3. Effects of T4 on mRNA abundance (RT-PCR) of pro-apoptotic *p21*, *c-fos*, and *c-jun* in human differentiated papillary (BHP 18-2) and follicular (FTC 236) thyroid carcinoma cells. Cells were treated in vitro for 24 h with resveratrol (RV) (10 µM) or T4 (10^{-7} M total hormone concentration, 10^{-10} M free hormone) or with both agents. T4 inhibited the expression of RV-induced pro-apoptotic genes and did not affect control *GAPDH* gene. *GAPDH*, glyceraldehyde 3-phosphate dehydrogenase. Reprinted with permission from Elsevier from Lin et al. [16].

Poorly differentiated or anaplastic thyroid carcinoma cells were not studied by Lin et al. in terms of possible responsiveness to T4.

3. Gene Expression in Thyroid Cancer Cells Exposed to Leptin

In the clinical setting of overweight, adipose tissue is expected to secrete leptin protein [27,28]. An endogenous anti-appetite factor, leptin has also been shown to support the growth of certain tumors, including papillary thyroid carcinoma, that express the leptin receptor [4]. There are a variety of other observations that link leptin and thyroid hormone together at cancer cells. Thyroid hormone may increase adipocyte secretion of leptin [29], and circulating leptin levels may be increased in papillary thyroid cancer patients [30]. Leptin variably modulates iodide uptake by thyroid cells [31]. Migration in vitro of papillary thyroid carcinoma cells is increased by leptin [32]. Finally, stimulation of epithelial-to-mesenchymal transition (EMT) is obtained with leptin [33] and with thyroid hormone [34], suggesting that both factors may support cancer metastasis.

Lin and co-workers have identified certain genes whose transcription is modulated in papillary thyroid carcinoma cells by leptin (Figure 4) [5]. Leptin and its derivative, OB3, both significantly reduce abundance of MMP9 mRNA in follicular thyroid cancer cells (Figure 4B), but do not affect expression of *MMP9* in papillary thyroid carcinoma cells (Figure 4A). In the latter cells, however, OB3 and leptin both reduce cell proliferation. Thus, leptin has thyroid cancer-type-specific actions on gene transcription. Such observations raise the possibility that body mass index with changes in endogenous leptin production may be associated with different clinical behaviors of papillary vs. follicular thyroid carcinomas.

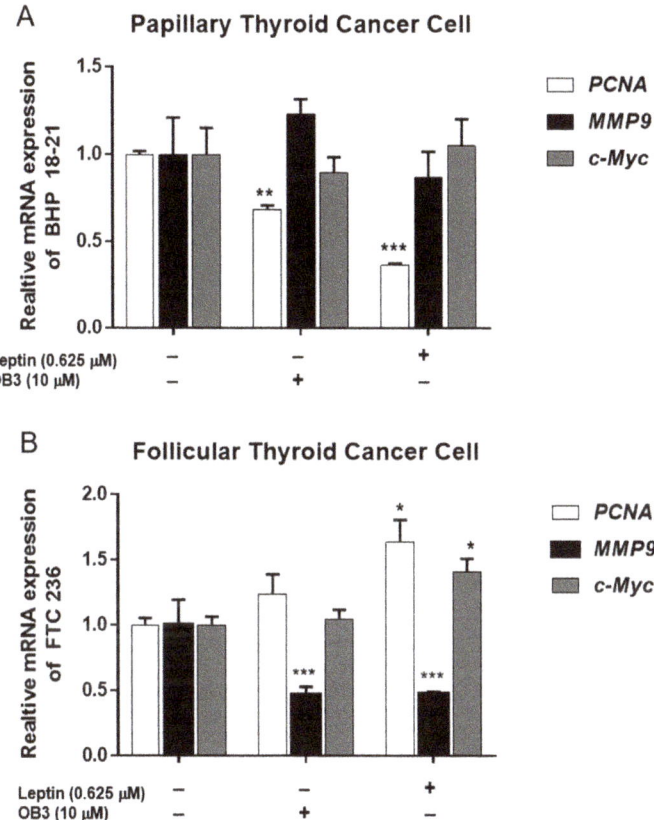

Figure 4. Effect of OB3 and leptin peptides on expression of genes relevant to invasion and cell proliferation in thyroid cancer cell lines. (**A**) Papillary and (**B**) follicular thyroid cancer cells were treated with either 0.625 µM leptin or 10 µM OB3 for 24 h. Cells were harvested, and total RNA was extracted. qPCR for *PCNA*, *MMP9* and *c-Myc* was conducted as described in Yang et al. [5]. Data were expressed as mean ± S.D. in triplicate. * $p < 0.05$, ** $p < 0.01$, *** $p < 0.001$, were compared with control.

4. Actions of Thyroid Hormone Analogues on Cells of Medullary Thyroid Carcinoma (MTC)

Medullary carcinoma originates in thyroid gland C cells, is thus distinct from papillary and follicular thyroid cancers and is an aggressive, non-TSH-dependent form of thyroid cancer. MTC may occur sporadically or conjunctively as a component of genetic multiple endocrine adenomatosis type 2 [35].

Gene expression that is subject to regulation in MTC cells by certain thyroid hormone analogues has been studied by Yalcin and co-workers [36]. In these studies, tetrac was the thyroid hormone analogue used to probe for thyroid hormone sensitivity of gene expression. Because tetrac, in various non-thyroidal cancer cells studied to-date, is anti-proliferative, pro-apoptotic, and anti-angiogenic [8,37]—the antithesis of T4 [19,21–24,38]—several implications of tetrac studies are clear. First, when it may be studied in the same cells, T4 is likely to have effects that are the direct opposite of tetrac and chemically modified tetrac. Tetrac is an antagonist of T4 at the integrin. Second, the panel of tetrac effects conveys the prospect of effectiveness as an anticancer agent. Third, the effects downstream on a) signal transduction and b) consequent gene expression of the $\alpha v \beta 3$ thyroid hormone receptor are extensive.

Acting on MCT cells grafted into the chick chorioallantoic membrane (CAM) model system, tetrac or tetrac analogues reduced tumor weight and tumor hemoglobin content—an index of angiogenesis—by more than 60% at 3 weeks [36]. This anti-angiogenic effect was then studied with q-PCR and RNA microarray in cultured MTC cells. Here, tetrac or a formulation of tetrac downregulated expression of vascular endothelial growth factor A (VEGFA) and upregulated anti-angiogenic thrombospondin 1 (THSB1) genes. The tumor shrinkage in the CAM studies reflected anti-angiogenesis, but in addition pro-apoptosis gene expression was observed. For example, significant increases in transcription of DFFA, FAF1 and CASP2 were induced by tetrac molecules. Thus, thyroid hormone analogues have access to control mechanisms via $\alpha v \beta 3$ for MCT angiogenesis- and apoptosis-relevant gene expression. Because tetrac is a specific inhibitor of the actions of T4 at integrin $\alpha v \beta 3$, we propose that T4 has actions in MCT cells that are anti-apoptotic, as has been shown to be the case in papillary and follicular thyroid cancer cells.

5. Discussion

Clinical activity of the various forms of thyroid carcinoma is largely a function of specific gene mutations and epigenetic changes that are the subjects of other papers in this issue of the journal. Endogenous TSH may be a trophic factor, particularly in differentiated thyroid cancers and, as pointed out above and elsewhere in this symposium, pharmacologic administration of T4 to suppress host pituitary TSH production may be therapeutically helpful. When differentiated thyroid carcinomas recur in the context of T4-conditioned suppression of TSH, we have suggested that the tumors are no longer TSH-dependent and, in fact, may be T4-dependent [3]. This possibility has not been systematically examined.

T4 is a growth factor for human carcinomas, including thyroid cancers, and a number of studies have concluded that a receptor for thyroid hormone analogues is involved on the extracellular domain of cancer cell integrin $\alpha v \beta 3$ [8,37,39,40]. Transduction of the T4 or other thyroid hormone analogue signal at the integrin results in the downstream modulation of transcription of a number of genes in a variety of cancers [8,37]. These genes are relevant to cancer cell division, to apoptosis, to invasiveness, and to tumor-relevant angiogenesis in a large panel of carcinomas of various organs. We have reviewed here the evidence for the trophic action of T4 on various forms of thyroid cancer. It is clear, however, that additional investigation is needed to confirm the extent of such action of T4. It is also of some importance to deal with the possibility that thyroid hormone analogues may act via integrin $\alpha v \beta 3$ to alter thyroid tumor radiosensitivity as they have been shown to do in other forms of cancers [41,42]. Also needed are studies that assess the possibility of effects of T4 on anaplastic thyroid carcinomas.

When differentiated thyroid carcinomas remain clinically active, despite full suppression of host TSH, we would suggest the possibility that the tumor is now T4-responsive [3]. A therapeutic option in this setting is induction of euthyroid hypothyroxinemia that we have tested clinically in a variety of advanced, T4-responsive (non-thyroid) cancers [43]. The limited genetic data we have reviewed in the current paper indicates a need for comparing genotypic information from differentiated, but now aggressive, thyroid cancers that (1) are and are not TSH-responsive and (2) are and are not T4-responsive in vitro. Genotyping of aspiration biopsies might then be useful in considering interruption of T4-suppression of TSH.

We have noted above that rT3—another thyroid hormone analogue thought to have little or no biological activity—is capable of stimulating cancer cell proliferation [11]. This proliferative effect has not yet been sought experimentally in differentiated thyroid carcinoma. However, the Type 3 deiodinase that generates rT3 from T4 [44] is present in papillary thyroid carcinoma cells [45].

Finally, we have also pointed out in the current review that leptin may be a trophic factor for papillary thyroid carcinoma, a form of cancer known to express the leptin receptor [5]. These interesting preclinical studies are of potential relevance to suboptimal clinical response of well-differentiated papillary thyroid cancer to TSH suppression in overweight patients. The genes whose expression was affected by leptin include those linked to angiogenesis and invasiveness.

Author Contributions: Conceptualization, P.J.D.; writing—original draft preparation, P.J.D.; writing—review and editing, P.J.D., H.-Y.L., A.H., and S.A.M. All authors have read and agreed to the published version of the manuscript.

Funding: This research received no external funding.

Acknowledgments: We thank Kelly A. Keating of the Pharmaceutical Research Institute for editing the manuscript and for constructing Figure 1.

Conflicts of Interest: Co-authors Davis and Mousa hold ownership in a pharmaceutical company that is developing tetrac-based anticancer agents. All other authors declare no conflict of interest.

References

1. Xing, M. Molecular pathogenesis and mechanisms of thyroid cancer. *Nat. Rev. Cancer* **2013**, *13*, 184–199. [CrossRef] [PubMed]
2. Roth, M.Y.; Witt, R.L.; Steward, D.L. Molecular testing for thyroid nodules: Review and current state. *Cancer* **2018**, *124*, 888–898. [CrossRef] [PubMed]
3. Davis, P.J.; Hercbergs, A.; Luidens, M.K.; Lin, H.Y. Recurrence of differentiated thyroid carcinoma during full tsh suppression: Is the tumor now thyroid hormone dependent? *Horm. Cancer* **2015**, *6*, 7–12. [CrossRef] [PubMed]
4. Celano, M.; Maggisano, V.; Lepore, S.M.; Sponziello, M.; Pecce, V.; Verrienti, A.; Durante, C.; Maranghi, M.; Lucia, P.; Bulotta, S.; et al. Expression of leptin receptor and effects of leptin on papillary thyroid carcinoma cells. *Int. J. Endocrinol.* **2019**, *2019*, 5031696. [CrossRef] [PubMed]
5. Yang, Y.C.; Chin, Y.T.; Hsieh, M.T.; Lai, H.Y.; Ke, C.C.; Crawford, D.R.; Lee, O.K.; Fu, E.; Mousa, S.A.; Grasso, P.; et al. Novel leptin OB3 peptide-induced signaling and progression in thyroid cancers: Comparison with leptin. *Oncotarget* **2016**, *7*, 27641–27654. [CrossRef]
6. Cheng, S.Y.; Leonard, J.L.; Davis, P.J. Molecular aspects of thyroid hormone actions. *Endocr. Rev.* **2010**, *31*, 139–170. [CrossRef]
7. Brent, G.A. Mechanisms of thyroid hormone action. *J. Clin. Investig.* **2012**, *122*, 3035–3043. [CrossRef]
8. Davis, P.J.; Goglia, F.; Leonard, J.L. Nongenomic actions of thyroid hormone. *Nat. Rev. Endocrinol.* **2016**, *12*, 111–121. [CrossRef]
9. Mousa, S.A.; Glinsky, G.V.; Lin, H.Y.; Ashur-Fabian, O.; Hercbergs, A.; Keating, K.A.; Davis, P.J. Contributions of thyroid hormone to cancer metastasis. *Biomedicines* **2018**, *6*, 89. [CrossRef]
10. Leonard, J.L.; Farwell, A.P. Thyroid hormone-regulated actin polymerization in brain. *Thyroid* **1997**, *7*, 147–151. [CrossRef]
11. Lin, H.Y.; Tang, H.Y.; Leinung, M.; Mousa, S.A.; Hercbergs, A.; Davis, P.J. Action of reverse T3 on cancer cells. *Endocr. Res.* **2019**, *44*, 148–152. [CrossRef] [PubMed]
12. Davis, P.J.; Mousa, S.A.; Cody, V.; Tang, H.Y.; Lin, H.Y. Small molecule hormone or hormone-like ligands of integrin αVβ3: Implications for cancer cell behavior. *Horm. Cancer* **2013**, *4*, 335–342. [CrossRef]
13. Cabanillas, M.E.; McFadden, D.G.; Durante, C. Thyroid cancer. *Lancet* **2016**, *388*, 2783–2795. [CrossRef]
14. Haugen, B.R.; Alexander, E.K.; Bible, K.C.; Doherty, G.M.; Mandel, S.J.; Nikiforov, Y.E.; Pacini, F.; Randolph, G.W.; Sawka, A.M.; Schlumberger, M.; et al. 2015 American Thyroid Association management guidelines for adult patients with thyroid nodules and differentiated thyroid cancer: The American Thyroid

Association Guidelines Task Force on Thyroid Nodules and Differentiated Thyroid Cancer. *Thyroid* **2016**, *26*, 1–133. [CrossRef]
15. Schmidbauer, B.; Menhart, K.; Hellwig, D.; Grosse, J. Differentiated thyroid cancer-treatment: State of the art. *Int. J. Mol. Sci.* **2017**, *18*, 1292. [CrossRef]
16. Lin, H.Y.; Tang, H.Y.; Shih, A.; Keating, T.; Cao, G.; Davis, P.J.; Davis, F.B. Thyroid hormone is a MAPK-dependent growth factor for thyroid cancer cells and is anti-apoptotic. *Steroids* **2007**, *72*, 180–187. [CrossRef]
17. Bergh, J.J.; Lin, H.Y.; Lansing, L.; Mohamed, S.N.; Davis, F.B.; Mousa, S.; Davis, P.J. Integrin αVβ3 contains a cell surface receptor site for thyroid hormone that is linked to activation of mitogen-activated protein kinase and induction of angiogenesis. *Endocrinology* **2005**, *146*, 2864–2871. [CrossRef]
18. Davis, P.J.; Shih, A.; Lin, H.Y.; Martino, L.J.; Davis, F.B. Thyroxine promotes association of mitogen-activated protein kinase and nuclear thyroid hormone receptor (TR) and causes serine phosphorylation of TR. *J. Biol. Chem.* **2000**, *275*, 38032–38039. [CrossRef]
19. Chen, Y.R.; Chen, Y.S.; Chin, Y.T.; Li, Z.L.; Shih, Y.J.; Yang, Y.S.H.; ChangOu, C.A.; Su, P.Y.; Wang, S.H.; Wu, Y.H.; et al. Thyroid hormone-induced expression of inflammatory cytokines interfere with resveratrol-induced anti-proliferation of oral cancer cells. *Food Chem. Toxicol.* **2019**, *132*, 110693. [CrossRef]
20. Hercbergs, A.; Mousa, S.A.; Leinung, M.; Lin, H.Y.; Davis, P.J. Thyroid hormone in the clinic and breast cancer. *Horm. Cancer* **2018**, *9*, 139–143. [CrossRef] [PubMed]
21. Lee, Y.S.; Chin, Y.T.; Shih, Y.J.; Nana, A.W.; Chen, Y.R.; Wu, H.C.; Yang, Y.S.H.; Lin, H.Y.; Davis, P.J. Thyroid hormone promotes β-catenin activation and cell proliferation in colorectal cancer. *Horm. Cancer* **2018**, *9*, 156–165. [CrossRef] [PubMed]
22. Shinderman-Maman, E.; Cohen, K.; Weingarten, C.; Nabriski, D.; Twito, O.; Baraf, L.; Hercbergs, A.; Davis, P.J.; Werner, H.; Ellis, M.; et al. The thyroid hormone-avb3 integrin axis in ovarian cancer: Regulation of gene transcription and MAPK-dependent proliferation. *Oncogene* **2016**, *35*, 1977–1987. [CrossRef] [PubMed]
23. Cohen, K.; Ellis, M.; Khoury, S.; Davis, P.J.; Hercbergs, A.; Ashur-Fabian, O. Thyroid hormone is a MAPK-dependent growth factor for human myeloma cells acting via αvβ3 integrin. *Mol. Cancer Res.* **2011**, *9*, 1385–1394. [CrossRef]
24. Davis, F.B.; Tang, H.Y.; Shih, A.; Keating, T.; Lansing, L.; Hercbergs, A.; Fenstermaker, R.A.; Mousa, A.; Mousa, S.A.; Davis, P.J.; et al. Acting via a cell surface receptor, thyroid hormone is a growth factor for glioma cells. *Cancer Res.* **2006**, *66*, 7270–7275. [CrossRef]
25. Lin, H.Y.; Chin, Y.T.; Nana, A.W.; Shih, Y.J.; Lai, H.Y.; Tang, H.Y.; Leinung, M.; Mousa, S.A.; Davis, P.J. Actions of L-thyroxine and nano-diamino-tetrac (Nanotetrac) on PD-L1 in cancer cells. *Steroids* **2016**, *114*, 59–67. [CrossRef]
26. Shih, A.; Davis, F.B.; Lin, H.Y.; Davis, P.J. Resveratrol induces apoptosis in thyroid cancer cell lines via a MAPK- and p53-dependent mechanism. *J. Clin. Endocrinol. Metab.* **2002**, *87*, 1223–1232. [CrossRef]
27. Zhang, Y.; Chua, S., Jr. Leptin function and regulation. *Compr. Physiol.* **2017**, *8*, 351–369.
28. Klok, M.D.; Jakobsdottir, S.; Drent, M.L. The role of leptin and ghrelin in the regulation of food intake and body weight in humans: A review. *Obes. Rev.* **2007**, *8*, 21–34. [CrossRef]
29. Yoshida, T.; Monkawa, T.; Hayashi, M.; Saruta, T. Regulation of expression of leptin mRNA and secretion of leptin by thyroid hormone in 3T3-L1 adipocytes. *Biochem. Biophys. Res. Commun.* **1997**, *232*, 822–826. [CrossRef]
30. Hedayati, M.; Yaghmaei, P.; Pooyamanesh, Z.; Zarif Yeganeh, M.; Hoghooghi Rad, L. Leptin: A correlated peptide to papillary thyroid carcinoma? *J. Thyroid Res.* **2011**, *2011*, 832163. [CrossRef]
31. de Oliveira, E.; Teixeira Silva Fagundes, A.; Teixeira Bonomo, I.; Curty, F.H.; Fonseca Passos, M.C.; de Moura, E.G.; Lisboa, P.C. Acute and chronic leptin effect upon in vivo and in vitro rat thyroid iodide uptake. *Life Sci.* **2007**, *81*, 1241–1246. [CrossRef]
32. Cheng, S.P.; Yin, P.H.; Chang, Y.C.; Lee, C.H.; Huang, S.Y.; Chi, C.W. Differential roles of leptin in regulating cell migration in thyroid cancer cells. *Oncol. Rep.* **2010**, *23*, 1721–1727. [PubMed]
33. Peng, C.; Sun, Z.; Li, O.; Guo, C.; Yi, W.; Tan, Z.; Jiang, B. Leptin stimulates the epithelialmesenchymal transition and proangiogenic capability of cholangiocarcinoma cells through the miR122/PKM2 axis. *Int. J. Oncol.* **2019**, *55*, 298–308. [PubMed]

34. Weingarten, C.; Jenudi, Y.; Tshuva, R.Y.; Moskovich, D.; Alfandari, A.; Hercbergs, A.; Davis, P.J.; Ellis, M.; Ashur-Fabian, O. The interplay between epithelial-mesenchymal transition (EMT) and the thyroid hormones-αvβ3 axis in ovarian cancer. *Horm. Cancer* **2018**, *9*, 22–32. [CrossRef]
35. Raue, F.; Frank-Raue, K. Multiple endocrine neoplasia type 2: 2007 update. *Horm. Res.* **2007**, *68*, 101–104. [CrossRef]
36. Yalcin, M.; Dyskin, E.; Lansing, L.; Bharali, D.J.; Mousa, S.S.; Bridoux, A.; Hercbergs, A.H.; Lin, H.Y.; Davis, F.B.; Glinsky, G.V.; et al. Tetraiodothyroacetic acid (tetrac) and nanoparticulate tetrac arrest growth of medullary carcinoma of the thyroid. *J. Clin. Endocrinol. Metab.* **2010**, *95*, 1972–1980. [CrossRef]
37. Davis, P.J.; Glinsky, G.V.; Lin, H.Y.; Leith, J.T.; Hercbergs, A.; Tang, H.Y.; Ashur-Fabian, O.; Incerpi, S.; Mousa, S.A. Cancer cell gene expression modulated from plasma membrane integrin αvβ3 by thyroid hormone and nanoparticulate tetrac. *Front. Endocrinol. (Lausanne)* **2014**, *5*, 240.
38. Meng, R.; Tang, H.Y.; Westfall, J.; London, D.; Cao, J.H.; Mousa, S.A.; Luidens, M.; Hercbergs, A.; Davis, F.B.; Davis, P.J.; et al. Crosstalk between integrin αvβ3 and estrogen receptor-α is involved in thyroid hormone-induced proliferation in human lung carcinoma cells. *PLoS ONE* **2011**, *6*, e27547. [CrossRef]
39. Latteyer, S.; Christoph, S.; Theurer, S.; Hones, G.S.; Schmid, K.W.; Fuhrer, D.; Moeller, L.C. Thyroxine promotes lung cancer growth in an orthotopic mouse model. *Endocr. Relat. Cancer* **2019**, *26*, 565–574. [CrossRef]
40. Cayrol, F.; Sterle, H.A.; Díaz Flaqué, M.C.; Barreiro Arcos, M.L.; Cremaschi, G.A. Non-genomic actions of thyroid hormones regulate the growth and angiogenesis of T cell lymphomas. *Front. Endocrinol.* **2019**, *10*, 63. [CrossRef]
41. Leith, J.T.; Mousa, S.A.; Hercbergs, A.; Lin, H.Y.; Davis, P.J. Radioresistance of cancer cells, integrin αvβ3 and thyroid hormone. *Oncotarget* **2018**, *9*, 37069–37075. [CrossRef] [PubMed]
42. Leith, J.T.; Hercbergs, A.; Kenney, S.; Mousa, S.A.; Davis, P.J. Activation of tumor cell integrin αvβ3 by radiation and reversal of activation by chemically modified tetraiodothyroacetic acid (tetrac). *Endocr. Res.* **2018**, *43*, 215–219. [CrossRef] [PubMed]
43. Hercbergs, A.; Johnson, R.E.; Ashur-Fabian, O.; Garfield, D.H.; Davis, P.J. Medically induced euthyroid hypothyroxinemia may extend survival in compassionate need cancer patients: An observational study. *Oncologist* **2015**, *20*, 72–76. [CrossRef] [PubMed]
44. Sibilio, A.; Ambrosio, R.; Bonelli, C.; De Stefano, M.A.; Torre, V.; Dentice, M.; Salvatore, D. Deiodination in cancer growth: The role of type III deiodinase. *Minerva Endocrinol.* **2012**, *37*, 315–327.
45. Romitti, M.; Wajner, S.M.; Ceolin, L.; Ferreira, C.V.; Ribeiro, R.V.; Rohenkohl, H.C.; Weber Sde, S.; Lopez, P.L.; Fuziwara, C.S.; Kimura, E.T.; et al. MAPK and SHH pathways modulate type 3 deiodinase expression in papillary thyroid carcinoma. *Endocr. Relat. Cancer* **2016**, *23*, 135–146. [CrossRef]

© 2020 by the authors. Licensee MDPI, Basel, Switzerland. This article is an open access article distributed under the terms and conditions of the Creative Commons Attribution (CC BY) license (http://creativecommons.org/licenses/by/4.0/).

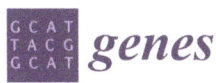

Article

VEGFA and *NFE2L2* Gene Expression and Regulation by MicroRNAs in Thyroid Papillary Cancer and Colloid Goiter

Leonardo P. Stuchi [1], Márcia Maria U. Castanhole-Nunes [1], Nathália Maniezzo-Stuchi [2], Patrícia M. Biselli-Chicote [1], Tiago Henrique [3], João Armando Padovani Neto [4], Dalisio de-Santi Neto [5], Ana Paula Girol [2], Erika C. Pavarino [1] and Eny Maria Goloni-Bertollo [1,*]

[1] Research Unit in Genetics and Molecular Biology—UPGEM, Faculty of Medicine of São José do Rio Preto—FAMERP, São José do Rio Preto 15090-000, Brazil; prado_leonardo@yahoo.com.br (L.P.S.); mcastanhole@gmail.com (M.M.U.C.-N.); patriciabiselli@yahoo.com.br (P.M.B.-C.); erika@famerp.br (E.C.P.)
[2] Padre Albino University Center—UNIFIPA, Catanduva, São Paulo 15809-144, Brazil; nmmbiomedica@hotmail.com (N.M.-S.); anapaula.girol@unifipa.com.br (A.P.G.)
[3] Laboratory of Molecular Markers and Bioinformatics, Department of Molecular Biology, Faculty of Medicine of São José do Rio Preto —FAMERP, São José do Rio Preto 15090-000, Brazil; henrique@famerp.br
[4] Department of Otolaryngology and Head and Neck Surgery, Faculty of Medicine of São José do Rio Preto —FAMERP, São José do Rio Preto 15090-000, Brazil; padovani.ja@gmail.com
[5] Pathological Anatomy Service, Hospital de Base, Foundation Regional Faculty of Medicine of São José do Rio Preto—FUNFARME, São José do Rio Preto 15090-000, Brazil; dalisius@gmail.com
* Correspondence: eny.goloni@famerp.br; Tel.: +55-17-3201-5720

Received: 27 May 2020; Accepted: 10 August 2020; Published: 19 August 2020

Abstract: Deregulation of VEGFA (Vascular Endothelial Growth Factor A) and NFE2L2 (Nuclear Factor (Erythroid-derived 2)-Like 2), involved in angiogenesis and oxidative stress, can lead to thyroid cancer progression. MiR-17-5p and miR-612 are possible regulators of these genes and may promote thyroid disorders. In order to evaluate the involvement of VEGFA, NFE2L2, hsa-miR-17-5p, and hsa-miR-612 in thyroid pathology, we examined tissue samples from colloid goiter, papillary thyroid cancer (PTC), and a normal thyroid. We found higher levels of VEGFA and NFE2L2 transcripts and the VEGFA protein in goiter and PTC samples than in normal tissue. In the goiter, miR-612 and miR-17-5p levels were lower than those in PTC. Tumors, despite showing lower *VEGFA* mRNA expression, presented higher VEGFA protein levels compared to goiter tissue. In addition, NRF2 (Nuclear Related Transcription Factor 2) protein levels in tumors were higher than those in goiter and normal tissues. Inhibition of miR-17-5p resulted in reduced NFE2L2 expression. Overall, both transcript and protein levels of NFE2L2 and VEGFA were elevated in PTC and colloid goiter. Hsa-miR-612 showed differential expression in PTC and colloid goiter, while hsa-miR-17-5p showed differential expression only in colloid goiter, suggesting that hsa-miR-17-5p may be a positive regulator of NFE2L2 expression in PTC.

Keywords: thyroid neoplasms; goiter; vascular endothelial growth factor A; NF-E2-related factor 2; microRNAs

1. Introduction

Colloid goiter is the most common disorder of the thyroid gland, even in non-endemic regions, and it is clinically detected in about 4% of individuals older than 30 years [1]. The presence of colloid goiter can indicate the beginning of malignant transformation of the thyroid leading to thyroid cancer [2,3].

Thyroid cancer is the most common endocrine neoplasia, accounting for about 1.7% of all cancer diagnoses worldwide [4], and it is the fifth most common type of cancer in women [5]. Papillary thyroid cancer (PTC) is the most common thyroid cancer, accounting for about 80% of diagnoses [6].

Angiogenesis plays a key role in the progression of cancer and the onset of metastases, as the newly formed blood vessels supply the nutrients and oxygen necessary for the maintenance of tumor growth [7]. VEGFA (Vascular Endothelial Growth Factor A) is the first angiogenic factor induced by hypoxia and promotes proliferation, budding, migration, and formation of the endothelial matrix [8]. Another important factor for angiogenesis is nuclear related transcription factor 2 (NRF2), encoded by the *NFE2L2* gene (*nuclear factor (erythroid-derived 2)-like 2*). NRF2 regulates the expression of antioxidant proteins in response to oxidative stress in various tissues [9]. Therefore, *VEGFA* and *NFE2L2* have been considered potential targets for new antiangiogenic therapies.

Gene expression can be regulated by microRNAs (miRNAs, miR), which control many cellular processes, including cell growth, differentiation, proliferation, and apoptosis [10]. Identification of the possible roles of miR-17-5p and miR-612 in the regulation of *NFE2L2* and *VEGFA* expression in PTC and colloid goiter can provide valuable insights for the development of strategies and drugs to inhibit tumor growth and also to restore sensitivity of tumors to chemotherapy.

In this study, we aimed to evaluate mRNA and protein levels of VEGFA and NFE2L2, as well as the expression patterns of miR-17-5p and miR-612 in human papillary thyroid cancer, colloid goiter, and normal thyroid tissues, and also to investigate the involvement of miR-17-5p and miR-612 in the regulation of *VEGFA* and *NFE2L2* expression in the thyroid papillary cancer cell line (TPC-1 line).

2. Materials and Methods

2.1. Specimens

Tumor and goiter tissue samples, along with adjacent tissues, as well as normal thyroid tissue samples were collected from 66 patients, as follows: 15 thyroid papillary cancer patients (13 females and 2 males), 15 goiter colloid patients (14 females and 1 male), and 6 patients with normal thyroid (4 females and 2 males). Tumor and goiter samples, along with adjacent tissue samples, were sent to the Pathology Service of Hospital de Base de São José do Rio Preto—SP for diagnosis and microdissection. The tumors were classified according to the parameters of "American Joint Committee for Cancer" (AJCC) [11]: tumor size (T), presence of nodal metastasis (N), and presence of distant metastasis (M). This study was approved by the Research Ethics Committee of the Medical School of São José do Rio Preto, FAMERP (No. 468.393).

2.2. Computer Prediction of miRs

miRs were selected in the DIANA-TarBase v7.0 database (http://diana.imis.athena-innovation.gr/DianaTools/index.php?r=tarbase/index), TargetScan (http://www.targetscan.org/vert_71) and mirDIP (http://ophid.utoronto.ca/mirDIP/). Two miRs with the highest score for regulation of *NFE2L2* and *VEGFA* were selected.

2.3. Expression of NFE2L2, VEGFA, miR-17-5p, and miR-612

RNA was extracted using the mirVana PARIS Kit (Applied Biosystems, Carlsbad, CA, USA). Complementary DNA (cDNA) from total RNA was synthesized using the High Capacity cDNA Archive Kit (Life Technologies, Carlsbad, CA, USA). The conversion of the miRs into cDNA was performed using the TaqMan-Micro RNA Reverse Transcription kit (Applied Biosystems).

Expression analyses of *NFE2L2* (Hs00975961_g1) and *VEGFA* (Hs00900055_m1), miR-17-5p (002308), and miR-612 (001579) were performed by quantitative real-time PCR (qPCR) using specific TaqMan probes (Thermo Fisher Scientific, Waltham, MA, USA) on the CFX 96 Real Time System

(Bio-Rad, Hercules, CA, USA). All reactions were performed in duplicates and included a contamination control. The genes *β-actin* (Hs01060665_g1) and *GAPDH* (Hs03929097_g1) were used as reference genes for normalization of *NFE2L2* and *VEGFA* expression data. The genes *RNU6B* (001093) and *RNU48B* (001006) were used for normalization of miR-17-5p and miR-612 expression data (Thermo Fisher Scientific). Relative quantification (RQ) of genes and miR expression in PTC and colloid goiter was calculated using the $2^{-\Delta\Delta Ct}$ method in relation to the normal tissues [12].

2.4. Quantification of Protein Expression in Tissue Samples

The proteins were extracted using the mirVana Paris Kit and Trizol Reagent (Applied Biosystems) and quantified using the BCA Protein Assay Kit (Abcam, Cambridge, United Kingdom).

Quantification of VEGFA protein in fresh tissue samples was performed using VEGFA Duo Set ELISA Kit (R&D Systems, Minneapolis, MN, USA) following the manufacturer's instruction. Immunohistochemistry was performed for analysis of NRF2 protein quantification. Briefly, after deparaffinization, the sections were rehydrated in a graded series of ethanol. The polyclonal rabbit anti-Nrf2 primary antibody (PA5-27882, Thermo Fisher Scientific) was used at a dilution of 1:100. After incubation, a biotinylated secondary antibody (Histostain-Plus IHC Kit, DAB, broad spectrum, 95-9943B, Invitrogen, Carlsbad, CA, USA) was used. The slides were incubated with streptavidin complex conjugated to peroxidase and 3,3'-diaminobenzidine (DAB 750118, Invitrogen) in the dark. For analysis of densitometry, the sections were photographed under a 40x objective (three fields per slide). For each sample, the cytoplasm and nucleus of epithelial cells were evaluated at 20 points equally distributed in the cytoplasm and 10 points in the nucleus.

2.5. Cell Line TPC-1 Culture

The TPC-1 cell line [13] derived from female papillary cancer was cultured in DMEM (Dulbecco's modified Eagle's medium, Cultilab, Campinas, Brazil), supplemented with 10% fetal bovine serum (Cultilab), 100 U/mL sodium penicillin, 100 mg/mL streptomycin (Cultilab), and 1% L-glutamine (Cultilab) at 37 °C in a 5% CO_2 incubator. The TPC-1 cell line authentication was performed by STR (Short Tandem Repeat) DNA typing profile using Gene Print 10 (Promega, Madison, WI, USA), ID 142738.

2.6. Transfection in the TPC-1 Cell Line

Transfection assays were conducted using mirVana™ inhibitor for miR-17-5p (MH12412, Thermo Scientific) and the mirVana™ miR-612 mimic (MC11461, Thermo Scientific) with Lipofectamine RNAiMAX (Invitrogen) following the manufacturer's instructions. Cells were cultured for 48 h in 100 µL of Opti-MEM serum-free medium (Invitrogen), 1 µL of Lipofectamine RNAiMAX (Invitrogen), and 10 mM of the inhibitor for miR-17-5p or the miR-612 mimic. RNA was extracted to verify the efficiency of transfection, using the respective positive and negative controls by qPCR.

2.7. Statistical Analyses

Statistical analyses were performed using GraphPad Prism software, version 6. The continuous data distribution was evaluated using D'Agostino and Pearson's normality test. The Wilcoxon signed rank test and the Mann–Whitney test were used to evaluate the gene expression data. The correlation between the expression of miRNAs and the genes was analyzed by Spearman's correlation. The Mann–Whitney test was used to evaluate the protein expression data. Values of $p < 0.05$ were considered significant.

3. Results

3.1. Characteristics of the Samples

The characteristics of the samples are summarized in Table 1.

Table 1. Characteristics of the collected samples.

Characteristics	Tumor	Goiter
Gender		
Female (F)	13 (86.7%)	14 (93.4%)
Male (M)	2 (13.3%)	1 (6.6%)
Age		
<45	F: 7 (46.6%); M: 1 (6.7%)	F: 6 (40%); M: 1 (6.7%)
≥45	F: 6 (40%); M: 1 (6.7%)	F: 8 (53.3%); M: 0 (-)
Tumor extent		
I	8 (53.4%)	
II-III	7 (46.6%)	
Nodal metastasis	2 (13.3%)	
Distant metastasis	2 (13.3%)	

3.2. Expression of VEGFA, NFE2L2, miR-17-5p, and miR-612 in Fresh Tissue Samples

Expression levels of *VEGFA*, *NFE2L2*, miR-17-5p, and miR-612 in the tumor tissues, colloid goiter, and their respective adjacent tissues were compared to those observed in the normal tissues. *VEGFA* and *NFE2L2* showed high expression levels in the tumor and goiter. MiR-17-5p and miR-612 did not exhibit differential expression in the tumor, but the expression levels of both miRs were reduced in the goiter (Table 2).

Table 2. Genes and miR expression in thyroid tumor and goiter in relation to normal thyroid tissue.

	Tumor				Goiter			
Gene	RQ Median	Min	Max	P	RQ Median	Min	Max	P
VEGFA	1.516	0.059	6.605	0.0125 *	20.010	8.595	32.260	<0.0001 *
NFE2L2	5.446	0.045	40.76	0.0061 *	23.380	0.278	68.780	0.0009 *
MicroRNAs								
miR-17-5p	0.206	0.007	3.305	0.094	0.099	0.006	0.879	<0.0001 *
miR-612	0.181	0.002	7.097	0.135	0.044	0.003	0.238	0.015 *

RQ, relative quantification; P, p value; *, Wilcoxon signed rank test.

VEGFA and *NFE2L2* also showed elevated expression in the tumor- and goiter-adjacent tissues. MiR-612 showed reduced expression in the tumor-adjacent tissue and in the goiter-adjacent tissue, whereas miR-17-5p showed reduced expression only in the goiter-adjacent tissue (Table 3).

Table 3. Gene and miR expression in tumor- and goiter-adjacent tissues in relation to normal thyroid tissue.

	Tumor-Adjacent Tissue				Goiter -Adjacent Tissue			
Gene	RQ Median	Min	Max	P	RQ Median	Min	Max	P
VEGFA	3.405	0.010	8.190	0.0023 *	20.720	13.820	55.970	<0.0001 *
NFE2L2	23.990	0.039	76.920	0.0149 *	15.870	2.417	83.740	<0.0001 *
MicroRNAs								
miR-17-5p	0.256	0.059	11.020	0.118	0.209	0.043	10.930	0.0448 *
miR-612	0.128	0.003	20.790	0.016 *	0.092	0.001	4.413	0.0131 *

RQ, relative quantification; P, p value; *, Spearman correlation.

Comparisons between the groups revealed that *VEGFA* gene expression was higher in the goiter than in the tumor (RQ median = 20.28 vs. 1.5; $p < 0.0001$) and also in the goiter-adjacent tissue than in the tumor-adjacent tissue (RQ median = 20.72 vs. 3.40, $p < 0.0001$) (Figure 1). No significant difference was detected in *NFE2L2* expression between the groups.

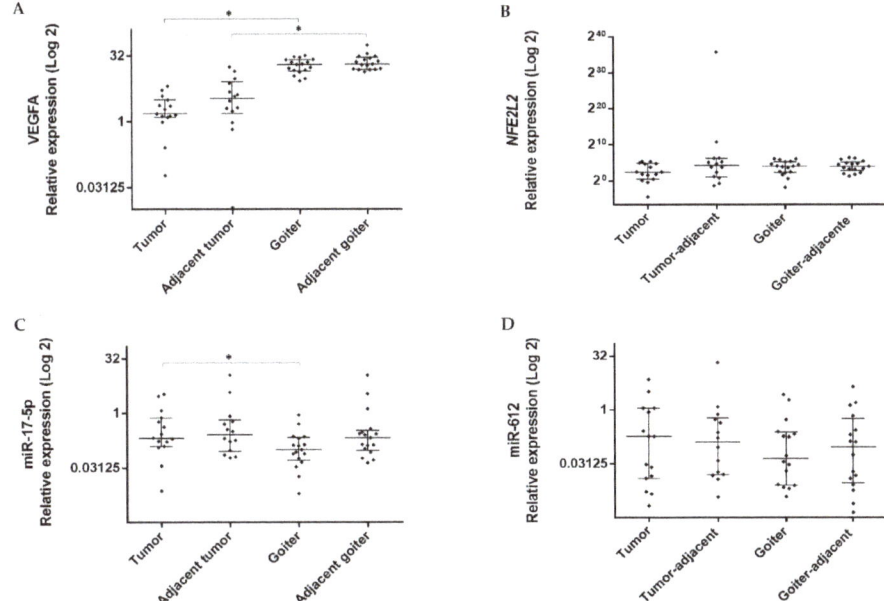

Figure 1. Expression levels of (**A**) *VEGFA* (*Vascular Endothelial Growth Factor A*), (**B**) *NFE2L2* (*Nuclear Factor (Erythroid-derived 2)-Like 2*), (**C**) miR-17-5p, and (**D**) miR-612 in tumor and goiter tissues and their respective adjacent tissues. Data are presented as median with interquartile range (25% percentile and 75% percentile). The relative expression value was Log2 transformed (y-axis). Calibrator (normal tissue) log RQ = 1. *, Statistically significant (panel A, Mann–Whitney, $p < 0.0001$; panel C, Mann–Whitney, $p = 0.033$).

Regarding miR expression, miR-17-5p expression was higher in the tumor than in the goiter (RQ median = 0.20 vs. 0.09; $p = 0.033$) (Figure 1). Expression of miR-612 did not differ significantly between the groups.

3.3. Correlation between Expression Levels of VEGFA, NFE2L2, miR-17-5p, and miR-612

There was a negative correlation in the tumor tissue between miR-612 and *VEGFA* expression, and between miR-612 and miR-17-5p and *NFE2L2* expression. In relation to the goiter, only miR-612 expression presented a negative correlation with *NFE2L2* expression (Table 4; Figure 2).

Table 4. Correlation between expression levels of *VEGFA* and *NFE2L2* and the miR-17-5p and miR-612 miRs in thyroid tumors and colloid goiter.

	Tumor				Goiter			
	VEGFA		NFE2L2		VEGFA		NFE2L2	
	R^2	P	R^2	P	R^2	P	R^2	P
miR17-5p	−0.411	0.130	−0.067	0.019 *	−0.118	0.653	−0.174	0.503
miR-612	−0.546	0.038 *	−0.679	0.007 *	−0.479	0.062	−0.724	0.002 *

R^2, correlation coefficient; P, p value; *, Spearman correlation.

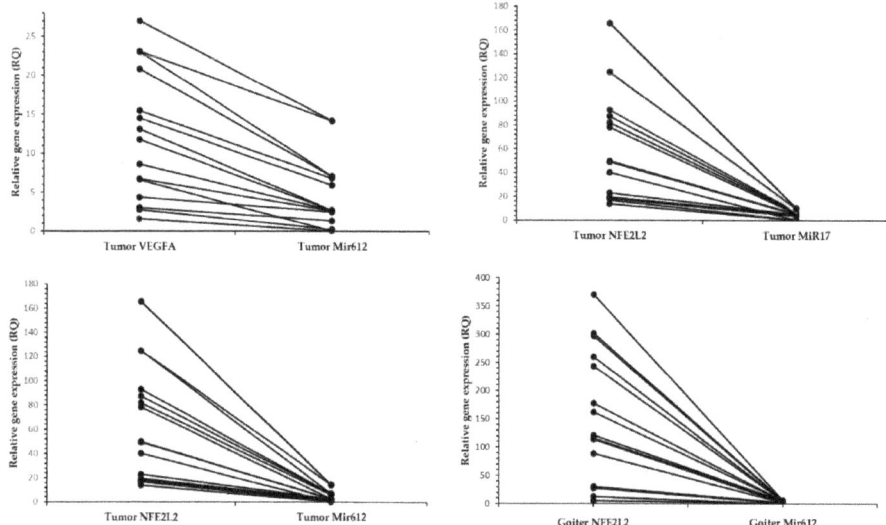

Figure 2. Relationship between relative expression levels of miRs and genes, showing high expression levels of genes and low expression levels of miRs. Each point represents an individual sample, for which the two gene expression levels are correspondingly connected. RQ, relative quantification.

3.4. Expression of VEGFA and NRF2 Proteins in Tissues

The protein levels of VEGFA were higher in the tumor compared to those in normal tissue ($p = 0.0009$), the goiter ($p = 0.0222$), and goiter-adjacent tissue ($p = 0.0003$). Tumor-adjacent tissue also presented elevated VEGFA protein levels compared to the normal tissues ($p = 0.0138$). The expression of VEGFA was upregulated in the goiter compared to the normal tissues ($p = 0.0397$) (Figure 3).

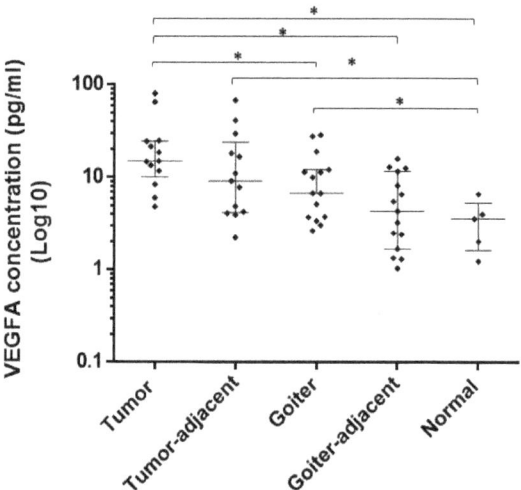

Figure 3. Protein expression of VEGFA in tumor, goiter, and normal tissue samples. VEGFA concentration was Log10 transformed (*y*-axis). Mann–Whitney test (* *p* value).

Expression of NRF2 protein in tumor tissues, colloid goiter, and normal tissues is shown in Figure 4. The cytoplasmic expression of NRF2 was higher in the tumor tissues compared to the normal tissues ($p < 0.0001$) and the goiter ($p < 0.0001$). In the nucleus, there was a stronger staining in the tumor tissue compared to the goiter tissue ($p < 0.0001$); no nuclear staining was observed in the normal thyroid tissues.

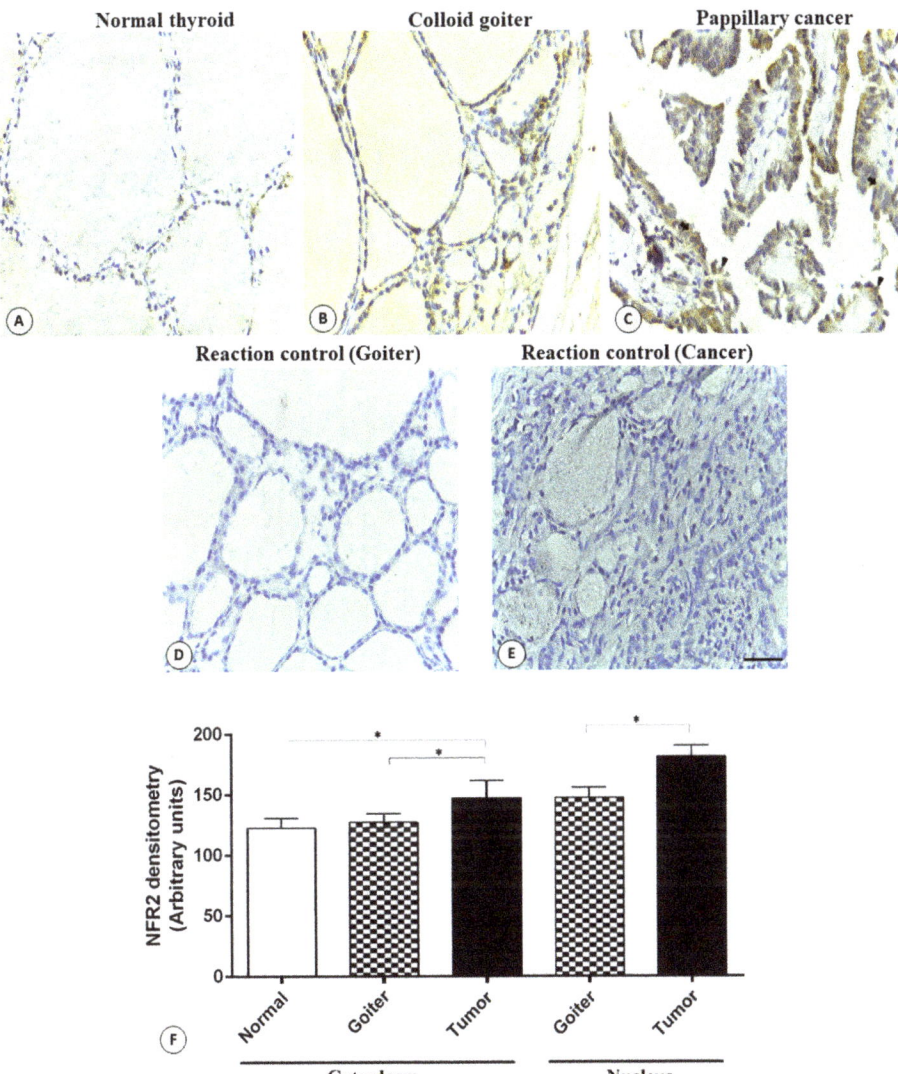

Figure 4. Expression of the NRF2 protein in the thyroid gland. Increased expression in the cytoplasm and nucleus in different tissues. (**A**) Normal thyroid tissue. (**B**) Colloid goiter. (**C**) Papillary thyroid cancer. (**D**) Negative controls of the goiter and (**E**) tumor. Section thickness, 5 μm; contra-staining, hematoxylin; scale bars, 20 μm. (**F**) Densitometric analysis of NRF2 quantification. The data represent the mean ± SEM of the densitometric index. *, $p < 0.0001$; bar size, 20 μm; arrows, cytoplasm; arrowhead, nucleus.

3.5. Superexpression Assay of miR-612 in the TPC-1 Cell Line

The transfection efficiency was checked on TPC-1 cells using the positive (mirVana™ miRNA Mimic miR-1 Positive Control, Life Technologies) and negative controls (mirVana ™ miRNA Mimic, Negative Control # 1, Life Technologies). Relative quantification ($2^{-\Delta\Delta Ct}$ method) of *TWF1* in cells treated with mirVana ™ miRNA Mimic miR-1 Positive Control revealed a 60% reduction in *TWF1* expression. The transfection with miR-612 did not show any significant difference in the expression of *VEGFA* and *NFE2L2* in the treated cells.

3.6. Inhibition Assay of miR-17-5p in the TPC-1 Cell Line

The transfection efficiency test for the inhibition assay using the positive control mirVana™ miRNA Inhibitor, let-7c positive control (Life Technologies) showed a 60% reduction in *HMGA2* expression. Transfection of miR-17-5p inhibitor into TPC-1 cells showed no difference in *VEGFA* expression, however, an approximately 73% inhibition in *NFE2L2* expression was noted (Figure 5).

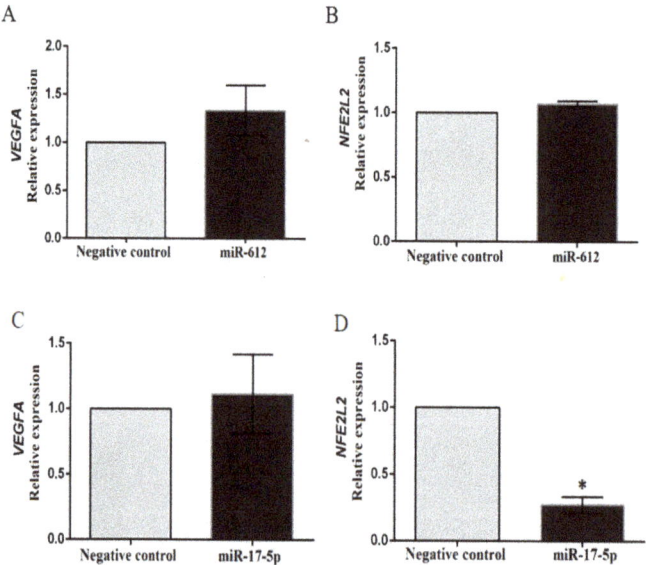

Figure 5. Results of the transfection assay on the TPC-1 cell line using mirVana™ miRNA Inhibitor for miR-17-5p, and mirVana™ miRNA Mimic for miR-612. *VEGFA* expression did not differ between cells transfected and non-transfected with miR-612 (**A**) and the inhibitor for miR-17-5p (**C**). *NFE2L2* expression did not differ between cells transfected and non-transfected with miR-612 (**B**); the inhibition of miR-17-5p resulted in approximately 73% inhibition of *NFE2L2* expression (**D**). *, approximately 73% inhibition of gene expression in relation to the negative control. Calibrator (negative control) log RQ = 1.

4. Discussion

We noted higher prevalence of cancer and goiter in females, which may be related to sex-differences. Porc et al. reported the first meta-analysis and revealed genetic factors that differentially affect thyroid function in males and females [14]. The present study shows that tissues affected by papillary thyroid cancer or colloid goiter, and their respective adjacent tissues present increased expression of *VEGFA* and *NFE2L2*, thereby providing evidence that vascularization and oxidative stress are imbalanced in these tissues. Corroborating with our results, earlier studies have shown that the expression of the *VEGFA* is higher in thyroid cancer, and may be crucial for the development of goiter, since the proliferation of endothelial cells precedes that of thyroid cells [15–18]. Studies have reported functional defects and increased expression of *NFE2L2* in the thyroid. Since this gene is involved in the maintenance of homeostasis against the physiologically generated oxidative stress during thyroid hormone synthesis, its dysregulation may contribute to the development of goiter as well as tumorigenesis of thyroid [19–21]. It is noteworthy that the expression levels of these genes increase according to the type and degree of thyroid cancer progression [15,22].

We also observed the elevated expression of these genes in the tissues adjacent to the tumor tissues in relation to the normal tissues. This indicates that the organ affected by cancer and goiter present altered physiology. This result highlights the importance of the normal tissue as a normalizer of the expression data in gene expression studies, since the tissue adjacent to tumor may not represent the normality of the tissue in true sense and, in fact, may present some of cellular alterations that precede these diseases. To the best of our knowledge, this is the first study to analyze the expression of *VEGFA* and *NFE2L2* in normal thyroid tissue for comparison with tumor tissue and goiter, as other studies have used adjacent non-malignant tissues for comparison.

The TCGA (The Cancer Genome Atlas Program) thyroid cancer dataset showed that VEGFA and NFE2L2 were highly expressed in normal tissue ($n = 59$) when compared with the primary tumor ($n = 505$). When analyzing the histology of thyroid tumors, it was found that, for VEGFA, the follicular thyroid papillary carcinoma ($n = 102$) was the closest to normal tissue, while the classical thyroid papillary carcinoma ($n = 358$), tall thyroid papillary carcinoma ($n = 36$) and others ($n = 9$) were down-regulated in relation to normal tissue. All NFE2L2 levels in cancer tissues were down-regulated in relation to normal tissue (Supplementary Material). These changes in expression levels in relation to normal tissue may be related to the sample number analyzed.

A comparison between tumor and colloid goiter and between tumor-adjacent tissue and goiter-adjacent tissue revealed a significantly higher expression of the *VEGFA* gene in the samples of colloid goiter and its adjacent tissue. This increase in the expression of the *VEGFA* gene in goiter may be due to several factors. Increasing endothelial cells is the first step in goiter formation, which exhibits levels of *VEGFA* expression similar to those observed in some types of thyroid cancer [23–25]. It is also worth mentioning that most of the papillary cancer samples analyzed in the present study presented early stages according to the TNM (Classification of Malignant Tumors) classification and that the levels of *VEGFA* gene expression increased according to the types and stages of tumor [15].

The expression of the *NFE2L2* gene did not differ significantly between the tissues. Evidence suggests that the difference between the tissues can be more effectively analyzed with the protein analysis of NRF2, because this protein occurs in degraded form in the normal tissue. In benign lesions, this degradation undergoes an imbalance, whereas in the tumor tissue it is possible to observe the migration of NRF2 to the nucleus, where this factor acts in response to oxidative stress, thus activating antioxidant enzymes [20,22].

In addition, the expression of miR-17-5p and miR-612 in PTC and colloid goiter samples and their respective adjacent tissues was also verified in comparison to the normal tissues, since these miRs may be related to the regulation of the genes investigated in this study. The results showed that miR-17-5p and miR-612 were not differentially expressed in tumor samples, and only miR-612 expression was reduced in tumor-adjacent tissue. In colloid goiter samples and goiter-adjacent tissue, the expression of these miRs was reduced.

MiR-17-5p has been studied in several cancers types, including thyroid cancer, and the results point to an elevated expression in tumor tissues [26–28]. However, the data available for PTC are not consistent with our findings. Zhao and Li (2015) observed significantly reduced miR-17-5p expression in thyroid papillary cancer samples in comparison to tumor-adjacent tissues [29]. The present study, however, did not find significant differences between the expression levels of miR-17-5p in tumor and non-tumor adjacent tissues, but a slight decrease in expression was observed; a larger sample size is required to reach a conclusion. Expression levels of miR-17-5p, on the other hand, were significantly reduced in the colloid goiter samples compared to those in normal tissues. No reports were found in the literature that corroborate or contrast with the findings of the present study. In the comparison between the tumor and goiter samples, we detected a significant increase in miR-17-5p expression in the tumor samples, indicating that even in initial stages the malignant tissue presents alteration of expression in comparison to the benign tissue.

Expression of miR-612 showed no significant difference in the tumor tissues, although its relative expression was low in these samples. However, in the tumor-adjacent tissues, colloid goiter and goiter-adjacent tissues, the expression of miR-612 was significantly reduced compared to that in the normal tissues. It was previously shown that this miR-612 exhibits reduced expression in colorectal cancer [30] and hepatocellular carcinoma (HCC), and that its expression is inversely proportional to tumor progression and aggressiveness in HCC [31]. Our results, deviating from the observations in HCC and colorectal cancer, suggest that the expression of this miR could increase with the degree of cellular alterations that lead to tumor formation, since the tumor-adjacent tissues and the goiter samples have significantly reduced expression of miR-612. As no data on miR-612 expression in PTC are available, further investigations are needed to clarify the role of miR-612 in this and other types of thyroid disorders.

The protein quantification results of VEGFA showed that the papillary cancer samples, the tumor-adjacent tissues, and the colloid goiter samples had increased expression of this protein in comparison to the normal tissues. In the comparisons between goiter and tissues adjacent to the goiter as well as between tumor tissues and tumor-adjacent tissues, no difference in VEGFA protein or transcript levels was observed. A comparison of VEGFA levels between tumor and goiter samples showed significantly higher expression in the tumor, a result suggesting a relation at the protein level opposite to that we observed in mRNA levels. This contradictory result between protein and transcript levels suggests that tumor tissue and goiter may present different mechanisms of post-transcriptional or post-translational regulation that could result in lower amounts of protein present in goiter.

In addition, VEGFA also participates in angiogenic stimulation through inhibition of PTEN (phosphatase and tensin homolog) expression. VEGFA triggers a cascade of signaling events, including activation of mitogen-activated protein kinase (MAPK) and phosphorylation of the Elk-1 transcription factor. These events promote an increase in the expression of members of the miR-17-92 group, repressing PTEN expression. It is known that the reduced expression of PTEN protein is associated with the development of thyroid cancer through the proliferation of endothelial cells. On the contrary, the genetic inactivation of miR-17-92 in endothelial cells results in peripheral vascular impairment in vivo [32,33]. These findings reinforce the importance of increased VEGFA protein in tumors and may explain the higher protein quantification observed in the tumor samples in comparison to the goiter.

Using the immunohistochemistry technique, it was possible to observe the presence of NRF2 protein, which is activated by oxidative stress, migrating from the cell cytoplasm to the nucleus where it exerts the function of transcription factor. The results observed in the present study showed that the labeling of this protein in the normal tissue is very weak (almost undetectable), and is observed only in the cytoplasm. In goiter, the labeling is intensified and it is already possible, in some cases, to observe the protein in the nucleus. Finally, in the tumor tissue, it is possible to see a strong labeling in the cytoplasm and nucleus. These data indicate that NRF2 protein is activated in PTC. Consistent with our data, Ziros et al. (2013) also observed the same labeling pattern in normal thyroid tissue, benign lesions and papillary cancer [20]. A recent study by Geng et al. (2017) indicates that the Nrf2 pathway is commonly activated in PTC and occasionally is activated in benign thyroid lesions, suggesting that prolonged activation of NRF2 and its elevated expression may contribute to the occurrence of nodular goiter and PTC [22]. The presence of strong labeling of the NRF2 protein in the nucleus of tumor cells reinforces its role in the regulation of antioxidant response related genes [34].

To obtain information about the possible miRs involved in the regulation of the *NFE2L2* and *VEGFA* genes, a database search was performed. Bioinformatic analysis revealed that miR-17-5p targets both *VEGFA* and *NFE2L2* genes. Previous studies have shown the interaction between miR-17 and *VEGFA* in the skin [35] and kidney [36,37]. The interaction of this miR with the *NFE2L2* gene was observed in the mammary gland [38]. The miR-612 showed regular expression of the *VEGFA* gene in the bone marrow [39]. To date, there are no studies that prove the interaction of miR-612 with *NFE2L2*; however, according to the databases consulted, miR-612 is predicted to regulate the *NFE2L2* gene.

After bioinformatic analysis, the inhibitor for miR-17-5p and the miR-612 mimic were selected for transfection into the TPC-1 cell line. The present study showed that inhibition of miR-17-5p resulted in reduced expression of the *NFE2L2* gene in the TPC-1 cells. The miR-17 cluster is known to reduce the expression of the *PTEN* gene. The *PTEN* gene is important for angiogenesis as it regulates genes such as *NFE2L2*. Rojo et al. (2014) showed that the inhibition of miR-17 increased *PTEN* expression, which in turn has a role in Nrf2 degradation pathway [40]. In the present study inhibition of miR-17-5p resulted in a decrease in *NFE2L2* expression, corroborating previous findings; however, the tissue expression data showed a negative correlation between the expression of this miR-17-5p and the *NFE2L2* gene. These contrasting results may reflect the participation of other active pathways in thyroid cancer that could influence *NFE2L2* expression. It is also worth mentioning the differences found between the findings of fresh tumor tissue samples and cell culture. Although in vitro studies are extremely important for functional studies, they cannot reproduce the complexity of the tumor microenvironment, nor can they mimic the different pathways involved in the disease progression.

The genes and miRs evaluated in this study present great potential for the diagnosis of colloid goiter and papillary cancer since they presented differential expression in these tissues. VEGFA and NRF2 proteins have been shown to be efficient in differentiating normal tissues from PTC. The negative regulation of miR-17-5p and miR-612 in colloid goiter also suggest the performance of these miRs as biomarkers for this thyroid condition.

Angiogenesis, oxidative stress, and deregulation of miRs are crucial for the development of thyroid disorders and cancer. The two genes evaluated in the present study can be possible therapeutic targets in the angiogenesis of thyroid disorders since the feedback between these genes and their regulation via miRs is of great importance for tumor development.

5. Conclusions

NFE2L2 and *VEGFA* genes and their protein products are widely expressed in PTC and colloid goiter. miR-612 has differential expression in the thyroid tumor and colloid goiter, while miR-17 is expressed only in the goiter. Hsa-miR-17-5p positively regulates the expression of the *NFE2L2* gene in PTC. This study showed the important relationship between miR-17-5p and *NFE2L2*, evidenced by the functional experiments. However, further studies regarding the influence of miR17-5p on *NFE2L2* and *VEGFA* and on the formation of new vessels in the colloid goiter and in PTC are needed.

Supplementary Materials: The following are available online at http://www.mdpi.com/2073-4425/11/9/954/s1, Figure S1: Expression of *VEGFA* in THCA based on Sample types; Figure S2: Expression of *VEGFA* in THCA based on Tumor histology; Figure S3: Expression of *NFE2L2* in THCA based on Sample types; Figure S4: Expression of *NFE2L2* in THCA based on Tumor histology; Table S1: P values for *VEGFA* gene comparisons; Table S2: P values for *NFE2L2* gene comparisons

Author Contributions: Conceptualization, L.P.S.; data curation, L.P.S. and P.M.B.-C.; formal analysis, L.P.S. and M.M.U.C.-N.; methodology, L.P.S., M.M.U.C.-N., N.M.-S., J.A.P.N., D.d.-S.N. and A.P.G.; resources, E.C.P. and E.M.G.-B.; supervision, E.M.G.-B.; bioinformatics analysis, T.H.; validation, L.P.S.; writing—original draft, L.P.S. and N.M.-S.; writing—review and editing, L.P.S. All authors have read and agreed to the published version of the manuscript.

Funding: This study was supported by a Grant from FAPESP- São Paulo Research Foundation (Grant 2015/04403-8), CNPq- National Council for Scientific and Technological Development, CAPES- Higher Education Improvement Coordination(Finance code 001) and Hospital de Base/FUNFARME-Foundation of Regional Faculty of Medicine of São José do Rio Preto.

Acknowledgments: TPC-1 cells were provided by Janete Cerutti, Federal University of São Paulo (UNIFESP).

Conflicts of Interest: The authors declare that the research was conducted in the absence of any commercial or financial relationships that could be construed as a potential conflict of interest.

References

1. Medeiros-Neto, G. Multinodular Goiter. In *Endotext*; De Groot, L.J., Chrousos, G., Dungan, K., Feingold, K.R., Grossman, A., Hershman, J.M., Koch, C., Korbonits, M., McLachlan, R., New, M., et al., Eds.; MDText.com, Inc.: Dartmouth, MA, USA, 2016.
2. Gandolfi, P.P.; Frisina, A.; Raffa, M.; Renda, F.; Rocchetti, O.; Ruggeri, C.; Tombolini, A. The incidence of thyroid carcinoma in multinodular goiter: Retrospective analysis. *Acta Bio Med. Atenei Parm.* **2004**, *75*, 114–117.
3. Campbell, M.J.; Seib, C.D.; Candell, L.; Gosnell, J.E.; Duh, Q.Y.; Clark, O.H.; Shen, W.T. The underestimated risk of cancer in patients with multinodular goiters after a benign fine needle aspiration. *World J. Surg.* **2015**, *39*, 695–700. [CrossRef]
4. Ferlay, J.; Shin, H.-R.; Bray, F.; Forman, D.; Mathers, C.; Parkin, D.M. Estimates of worldwide burden of cancer in 2008: GLOBOCAN 2008. *Int. J. Cancer* **2010**, *127*, 2893–2917. [CrossRef]
5. Jemal, A. Cancer Statistics, 2010. *CA Cancer J. Clin.* **2011**, *61*, 133. [CrossRef]
6. DeLellis, R.A. *Pathology and Genetics of Tumours of Endocrine Organs*; IARC Press: Lyon, France, 2004; p. 320.
7. Biselli-Chicote, P.M.; Oliveira, A.R.; Pavarino, E.C.; Goloni-Bertollo, E.M. VEGF gene alternative splicing: Pro- and anti-angiogenic isoforms in cancer. *J. Cancer Res. Clin. Oncol.* **2012**, *138*, 363–370. [CrossRef]
8. Ferrara, N.; Gerber, H.P.; LeCouter, J. The biology of VEGF and its receptors. *Nat. Med.* **2003**, *9*, 669–676. [CrossRef]
9. Sporn, M.B.; Liby, K.T. NRF2 and cancer: The good, the bad and the importance of context. *Nat. Rev. Cancer* **2012**, *12*, 564–571. [CrossRef]
10. Bartel, D.P. MicroRNAs: Genomics, biogenesis, mechanism, and function. *Cell* **2004**, *116*, 281–297. [CrossRef]
11. Greene, F.L. The American Joint Committee on Cancer: Updating the strategies in cancer staging. *Bull. Am. Coll. Surg.* **2002**, *87*, 13–15. [PubMed]
12. Pfaffl, M.W. A new mathematical model for relative quantification in real-time RT-PCR. *Nucleic Acids Res.* **2001**, *29*, e45. [CrossRef] [PubMed]
13. Tanaka, J.; Ogura, T.; Sato, H.; Hatano, M. Establishment and biological characterization of an in vitro human cytomegalovirus latency model. *Virology* **1987**, *161*, 62–72. [CrossRef]
14. Porcu, E.; Medici, M.; Pistis, G.; Volpato, C.B.; Wilson, S.G.; Cappola, A.R.; Bos, S.D.; Deelen, J.; den Heijer, M.; Freathy, R.M.; et al. A meta-analysis of thyroid-related traits reveals novel loci and gender-specific differences in the regulation of thyroid function. *PLoS Genet.* **2013**, *9*, e1003266. [CrossRef] [PubMed]
15. Salajegheh, A.; Pakneshan, S.; Rahman, A.; Dolan-Evans, E.; Zhang, S.; Kwong, E.; Gopalan, V.; Lo, C.Y.; Smith, R.A.; Lam, A.K. Co-regulatory potential of vascular endothelial growth factor-A and vascular endothelial growth factor-C in thyroid carcinoma. *Hum. Pathol.* **2013**, *44*, 2204–2212. [CrossRef] [PubMed]
16. Salajegheh, A.; Vosgha, H.; Rahman, M.A.; Amin, M.; Smith, R.A.; Lam, A.K. Interactive role of miR-126 on VEGF-A and progression of papillary and undifferentiated thyroid carcinoma. *Hum. Pathol.* **2016**, *51*, 75–85. [CrossRef] [PubMed]
17. Malkomes, P.; Oppermann, E.; Bechstein, W.O.; Holzer, K. Vascular endothelial growth factor–marker for proliferation in thyroid diseases? *Exp. Clin. Endocrinol. Diabetes* **2013**, *121*, 6–13. [CrossRef]
18. Mohamad Pakarul Razy, N.H.; Wan Abdul Rahman, W.F.; Win, T.T. Expression of Vascular Endothelial Growth Factor and Its Receptors in Thyroid Nodular Hyperplasia and Papillary Thyroid Carcinoma: A Tertiary Health Care Centre Based Study. *Asian Pac. J. Cancer Prev. APJCP* **2019**, *20*, 277–282. [CrossRef] [PubMed]
19. Martinez, V.D.; Vucic, E.A.; Pikor, L.A.; Thu, K.L.; Hubaux, R.; Lam, W.L. Frequent concerted genetic mechanisms disrupt multiple components of the NRF2 inhibitor KEAP1/CUL3/RBX1 E3-ubiquitin ligase complex in thyroid cancer. *Mol. Cancer* **2013**, *12*, 124. [CrossRef]
20. Ziros, P.G.; Manolakou, S.D.; Habeos, I.G.; Lilis, I.; Chartoumpekis, D.V.; Koika, V.; Soares, P.; Kyriazopoulou, V.E.; Scopa, C.D.; Papachristou, D.J.; et al. Nrf2 is commonly activated in papillary thyroid carcinoma, and it controls antioxidant transcriptional responses and viability of cancer cells. *J. Clin. Endocrinol. Metab.* **2013**, *98*, E1422–E1427. [CrossRef]
21. Teshiba, R.; Tajiri, T.; Sumitomo, K.; Masumoto, K.; Taguchi, T.; Yamamoto, K. Identification of a KEAP1 germline mutation in a family with multinodular goitre. *PLoS ONE* **2013**, *8*, e65141. [CrossRef]
22. Geng, W.J.; Shan, L.B.; Wang, J.S.; Li, N.; Wu, Y.M. Expression and significance of Nrf2 in papillary thyroid carcinoma and thyroid goiter. *Zhonghua Zhong Liu Za Zhi [Chin. J. Oncol.]* **2017**, *39*, 367–368. [CrossRef]

23. Ramsden, J.D. Angiogenesis in the thyroid gland. *J. Endocrinol.* **2000**, *166*, 475–480. [CrossRef] [PubMed]
24. Klein, M.; Catargi, B. VEGF in physiological process and thyroid disease. *Annales d Endocrinologie* **2007**, *68*, 438–448. [CrossRef] [PubMed]
25. Wolinski, K.; Stangierski, A.; Szczepanek-Parulska, E.; Gurgul, E.; Budny, B.; Wrotkowska, E.; Biczysko, M.; Ruchala, M. VEGF-C Is a Thyroid Marker of Malignancy Superior to VEGF-A in the Differential Diagnostics of Thyroid Lesions. *PLoS ONE* **2016**, *11*, e0150124. [CrossRef] [PubMed]
26. Gu, R.; Huang, S.; Huang, W.; Li, Y.; Liu, H.; Yang, L.; Huang, Z. MicroRNA-17 family as novel biomarkers for cancer diagnosis: A meta-analysis based on 19 articles. *Tumour Biol. J. Int. Soc. Oncodevelopmental Biol. Med.* **2016**, *37*, 6403–6411. [CrossRef] [PubMed]
27. Yuan, Z.M.; Yang, Z.L.; Zheng, Q. Deregulation of microRNA expression in thyroid tumors. *J. Zhejiang Univ. Sci. B* **2014**, *15*, 212–224. [CrossRef]
28. Yang, Z.; Yuan, Z.; Fan, Y.; Deng, X.; Zheng, Q. Integrated analyses of microRNA and mRNA expression profiles in aggressive papillary thyroid carcinoma. *Mol. Med. Rep.* **2013**, *8*, 1353–1358. [CrossRef]
29. Zhao, S.; Li, J. Sphingosine-1-phosphate induces the migration of thyroid follicular carcinoma cells through the microRNA-17/PTK6/ERK1/2 pathway. *PLoS ONE* **2015**, *10*, e0119148. [CrossRef]
30. Sheng, L.; He, P.; Yang, X.; Zhou, M.; Feng, Q. miR-612 negatively regulates colorectal cancer growth and metastasis by targeting AKT2. *Cell Death Dis.* **2015**, *6*, e1808. [CrossRef]
31. Tao, Z.H.; Wan, J.L.; Zeng, L.Y.; Xie, L.; Sun, H.C.; Qin, L.X.; Wang, L.; Zhou, J.; Ren, Z.G.; Li, Y.X.; et al. miR-612 suppresses the invasive-metastatic cascade in hepatocellular carcinoma. *J. Exp. Med.* **2013**, *210*, 789–803. [CrossRef]
32. Fiedler, J.; Thum, T. New Insights Into miR-17-92 Cluster Regulation and Angiogenesis. *Circ. Res.* **2016**, *118*, 9–11. [CrossRef]
33. Chamorro-Jorganes, A.; Lee, M.Y.; Araldi, E.; Landskroner-Eiger, S.; Fernandez-Fuertes, M.; Sahraei, M.; Quiles Del Rey, M.; van Solingen, C.; Yu, J.; Fernandez-Hernando, C.; et al. VEGF-Induced Expression of miR-17-92 Cluster in Endothelial Cells Is Mediated by ERK/ELK1 Activation and Regulates Angiogenesis. *Circ. Res.* **2016**, *118*, 38–47. [CrossRef] [PubMed]
34. Zhou, S.; Ye, W.; Zhang, M.; Liang, J. The effects of nrf2 on tumor angiogenesis: A review of the possible mechanisms of action. *Crit. Rev. Eukaryot. Gene Expr.* **2012**, *22*, 149–160. [CrossRef] [PubMed]
35. Greenberg, E.; Hajdu, S.; Nemlich, Y.; Cohen, R.; Itzhaki, O.; Jacob-Hirsch, J.; Besser, M.J.; Schachter, J.; Markel, G. Differential regulation of aggressive features in melanoma cells by members of the miR-17-92 complex. *Open Biol.* **2014**, *4*, 140030. [CrossRef] [PubMed]
36. Ye, W.; Lv, Q.; Wong, C.K.; Hu, S.; Fu, C.; Hua, Z.; Cai, G.; Li, G.; Yang, B.B.; Zhang, Y. The effect of central loops in miRNA:MRE duplexes on the efficiency of miRNA-mediated gene regulation. *PLoS ONE* **2008**, *3*, e1719. [CrossRef]
37. Karginov, F.V.; Hannon, G.J. Remodeling of Ago2-mRNA interactions upon cellular stress reflects miRNA complementarity and correlates with altered translation rates. *Genes Dev.* **2013**, *27*, 1624–1632. [CrossRef]
38. Pillai, M.M.; Gillen, A.E.; Yamamoto, T.M.; Kline, E.; Brown, J.; Flory, K.; Hesselberth, J.R.; Kabos, P. HITS-CLIP reveals key regulators of nuclear receptor signaling in breast cancer. *Breast Cancer Res. Treat.* **2014**, *146*, 85–97. [CrossRef]
39. Baraniskin, A.; Kuhnhenn, J.; Schlegel, U.; Chan, A.; Deckert, M.; Gold, R.; Maghnouj, A.; Zollner, H.; Reinacher-Schick, A.; Schmiegel, W.; et al. Identification of microRNAs in the cerebrospinal fluid as marker for primary diffuse large B-cell lymphoma of the central nervous system. *Blood* **2011**, *117*, 3140–3146. [CrossRef]
40. Rojo, A.I.; Rada, P.; Mendiola, M.; Ortega-Molina, A.; Wojdyla, K.; Rogowska-Wrzesinska, A.; Hardisson, D.; Serrano, M.; Cuadrado, A. The PTEN/NRF2 axis promotes human carcinogenesis. *Antioxid. Redox Signal.* **2014**, *21*, 2498–2514. [CrossRef]

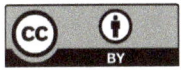

© 2020 by the authors. Licensee MDPI, Basel, Switzerland. This article is an open access article distributed under the terms and conditions of the Creative Commons Attribution (CC BY) license (http://creativecommons.org/licenses/by/4.0/).

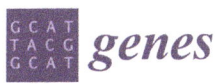

Article

Biomarkers, Master Regulators and Genomic Fabric Remodeling in a Case of Papillary Thyroid Carcinoma

Dumitru A. Iacobas

Personalized Genomics Laboratory, CRI Center for Computational Systems Biology, Roy G Perry College of Engineering, Prairie View A&M University, Prairie View, TX 77446, USA; daiacobas@pvamu.edu;
Tel.: +1-936-261-9926

Received: 1 August 2020; Accepted: 1 September 2020; Published: 2 September 2020

Abstract: Publicly available (own) transcriptomic data have been analyzed to quantify the alteration in functional pathways in thyroid cancer, establish the gene hierarchy, identify potential gene targets and predict the effects of their manipulation. The expression data have been generated by profiling one case of papillary thyroid carcinoma (PTC) and genetically manipulated BCPAP (papillary) and 8505C (anaplastic) human thyroid cancer cell lines. The study used the genomic fabric paradigm that considers the transcriptome as a multi-dimensional mathematical object based on the three independent characteristics that can be derived for each gene from the expression data. We found remarkable remodeling of the thyroid hormone synthesis, cell cycle, oxidative phosphorylation and apoptosis pathways. Serine peptidase inhibitor, Kunitz type, 2 (*SPINT2*) was identified as the Gene Master Regulator of the investigated PTC. The substantial increase in the expression synergism of *SPINT2* with apoptosis genes in the cancer nodule with respect to the surrounding normal tissue (NOR) suggests that *SPINT2* experimental overexpression may force the PTC cells into apoptosis with a negligible effect on the NOR cells. The predictive value of the expression coordination for the expression regulation was validated with data from 8505C and BCPAP cell lines before and after lentiviral transfection with *DDX19B*.

Keywords: 8505C cell line; apoptosis; BCPAP cell line; BRAF; CFLAR; IL6; oxidative phosphorylation; SPINT2; thyroid hormone synthesis; weighted pathway regulation

---

1. Introduction

Thyroid cancer (**TC**) has a lower incidence and mortality rate compared to other malignancies. Still, in 2020 in the USA, 52,440 new cases (12,270 men and 40,170 women) are expected to be added. Although TC affects over three times more women than men, the number of deaths (2180) is practically equally distributed between the two sexes (1040 men and 1140 women) [1]. There are four major types of thyroid cancers: papillary (hereafter denoted as **PTC**, 70–80% of total cases), follicular (**FTC**, 10–15%), medullary (**MTC**, ~2%) and anaplastic (**APC**, ~2%). PTC, FTC and MTC are composed of well-differentiated cells and are treatable, while APC is undifferentiated and has a poor prognosis [2].

Considerable effort has been invested in recent decades to identify DNA mutations and the oncogenes (which turn on) and tumor suppressor factors (which turn off) that are responsible for triggering TC. The 25.0 release (22 July 2020) of the Genomic Data Commons Data Portal [3] includes 11,128 confirmed mutations detected on 13,564 genes sequenced from 1440 (553 male and 887 female) TC cases. The most frequently mutated gene reported in the portal is *BRAF* (B-Raf proto-oncogene, serine/threonine kinase), with up to 10 mutations identified in 20.56% of cases. Further down in terms of mutation frequency are: *NRAS* (neuroblastoma RAS viral (v-ras) oncogene homolog) with two mutations in 2.71% of cases, *TTN* (titin), with a total of 40 mutations in 2.29% of cases, and *TG* (thyroglobulin), with a total of 26 mutations in 1.67% of cases [3]. For most genes, the portal [3] shows the specific types and locations of the mutations and the cancer form(s) where these mutations were found. However, there is no bi-univocal correspondence between cancer forms and mutated genes: each cancer was associated with numerous mutated genes and mutations of the same gene were identified in several forms of cancer. How many mutated genes does one need in order to decide upon the right form of cancer? Are there exclusive combinations of mutations for a particular form of cancer and only for that form? If present, the number of the affected genes should be large enough to avoid any overlap with other form of cancer. Although the incidence of each particular mutation in the explored cohort of patients is known, it is impossible to determine the predictive values of combinations of mutated genes because for more than three genes the number of possibilities ($\geq 2.3 \times 10^{11}$) exceeds the human population of the Earth. Even though one can determine via conditioned probabilities (actual conditioned frequencies) the chance of finding the same combination of mutations in other persons, the diagnostic value is very poor. Moreover, one should not forget that the mutations were identified with respect to a reference human genome obtained by averaging the DNA sequence results from a large number of healthy individuals regardless of race, sex, age, environmental conditions, etc. However, even among genomes of healthy individuals there are 0.1% (i.e., ~3mln nucleotides) differences (0.6% when considering indels) [4].

There are several commercially available gene assays used for the preoperative diagnostic and classification of TCs (e.g., [5,6]). Recently, Foundation Medicine [7] compiled a list of 310 genes with full coding exonic regions for the detection of substitutions, insertion–deletions and copy-number alterations. An additional list of the same Foundation contains 36 genes with intronic regions useful for the detection of gene rearrangements (one gene with a promoter region and one non-coding RNA gene) [7]. For all these assays, the question is how many and what genes should be mutated/regulated to assign an accurate diagnostic? Most importantly, how did the researchers determine the predictive values of each combination of genes? In [7], there are 346 combinations of one gene, 59,685 of two, 6,843,880 combinations of three, 587 million of four and over 40 billion of five and more. Therefore, for practical reasons, only the most relevant three biomarkers, at most, are currently used, which considerably limits the diagnostic accuracy.

While the diagnostic value of mutations and/or regulations is doubtful, what about their use for therapeutic purposes? Is restoring the normal sequence/expression level of one biomarker enough to cure the cancer? Considering that the "trusted" biomarkers were selected from the genes with the most frequently altered sequence and/or expression level in large populations, this means that they are less protected by the cellular homeostatic mechanisms. The cells are supposed to invest energy to protect the sequence and expression level of genes, critical for their survival, proliferation, and integration in multicellular structures. The low level of protection indicates that biomarkers are minor players, and therefore the restoration of their structure/expression level may be of little consequence to the cancer cells.

While we do not see a genomic solution for the cancer diagnostic at present, we believe that our Gene Master Regulator (**GMR**) approach [8,9] is a reasonable alternative to the actual biomarker-oriented gene therapy. The GMR of a particular cell phenotype is the gene whose highly protected sequence/expression by the cellular homeostatic mechanisms regulates major functional pathways through expression coordination with many of their genes. In our cancer genomic studies [8–10], we found that the GMR of the cancer nodule is very low in the gene hierarchy of the surrounding cancer-free tissue of the tumor. For this reason, manipulation of the GMR's expression is expected to selectively destroy cancer cells without affecting the normal ones much.

In this report, we analyze previously published transcriptomic data [8] to quantify the cancer-related remodeling of major functional pathways in the PTC nodule with respect to the normal tissue of the resection margins (**NOR**) of a surgically removed thyroid tumor. The Gene Commanding Height (**GCH**) hierarchy and the GMRs are determined in both PTC and NOR, and the potential regulations of the apoptosis genes in response to the cancer GMR expression manipulation are predicted. The GCH scores of the top genes are compared to those of the most mutated genes in TC as well as those of the usually considered cancer biomarkers. Transcriptomic profiles of two standard TC cell lines before and after stable transfection with a gene were used to determine the predictive value of the expression coordination with that gene in untreated cells for the regulation in treated ones. The analysis presented here was derived from the Genomic Fabric Paradigm (GFP) that assigns three independent measures to each gene and considers the transcriptome as a multi-dimensional mathematical object [11].

2. Materials and Methods

2.1. Gene Expression Data

We used gene expression data from one case of papillary thyroid carcinoma, pathological stage pT3NOMx, deposited in the Gene Expression Omnibus (GEO) of the National Center for Biotechnology Information (NCBI) [12] as GSE97001. In that study, the quarters of the most homogeneous 20-mm^3 part of the frozen unilateral, single, 32.0-mm PTC nodule and four small pieces from the NOR of the same gland from the same patient were profiled separately. Thus, we got data from four biological replicas of each region. Since each human is subjected to a unique set of transcriptome-regulating factors (race, sex, age, medical history, environmental conditions, exposure to stress and toxins, etc.), the normal tissue surrounding the cancer nodule is a far better reference than tissues from other healthy persons. Expression values were normalized iteratively to the median of all quantifiable genes in all samples and transcript abundances were presented as multiples of the expression level of the median gene in each region.

Transcriptomic data from the surgically removed tumor were compared to the gene expression profiles of two standard human thyroid cancer cell lines: BCPAP (papillary) and 8505C (anaplastic) deposited as GSE97002. We determined the predictive value of the coordination analysis in untreated cells for the expression regulation in treated ones by comparing the transcriptomic profiles of these cell lines before and after stable transfection with *DDX19B, NEMP1, PANK2* and *UBALD1*. The results of transfection with DEAD (Asp-Glu-Ala-Asp) box polypeptide 19B (*DDX17B*) were collected from GSE97028, those for nuclear envelope integral membrane protein 1 (*NEMP1*) from GSE97031, for pantothenate kinase 2 (*PANK2*) from GSE97030 and for UBA-like domain containing 1 (*UBALD1*) from GSE97427. Although alterations of *DDX19B* [13], *NEMP1* [14] and *PANK2* [15] were linked to some forms of cancer by other authors, these genes were selected only because their different GCH scores in the two cell lines made them suitable to validate the GMR approach [8,9].

2.2. Single-Gene Transcriptomic Quantifiers

2.2.1. Biological Replicas, Profiling Redundancy and Average Expression Level

The four biological replicas experimental design provided for every single gene in each region three independent measures: (i) average expression level, (ii) expression variation and (iii) expression coordination with each other gene [16]. We used these three measures and combinations of them to establish the gene hierarchies and characterize the contribution of each gene to the cancer-related reorganization of the thyroid transcriptome.

The Agilent two-color expression microarrays used in the analyzed experiment redundantly probed the genes with various number of spots from 1 to 20 (as for *MIEF1* = mitochondrial elongation factor 1) and *SRRT* = serrate, RNA effector molecule). Therefore, for each gene "i", we computed the average expression level over the group of R_i spots redundantly probing the same transcript of the average expression levels measured by spot "k" across the biological replicas.

$$\mu_i^{(NOR/PTC)} = \frac{1}{R_i}\sum_{k=1}^{R_i}\mu_{i,k}^{(NOR/PTC)} = \frac{1}{R_i}\sum_{k=1}^{R_i}\left(\frac{1}{4}\sum_{j=1}^{4}a_{i,k,j}^{(NOR/PTC)}\right), \text{ where:} \quad (1)$$

$a_{i,k,j}^{(NOR/PTC)}$ = expression level of gene "i" probed by spot "k" on biological replica "j"

2.2.2. Expression Variation

Because of the probing redundancy, instead of the coefficient of variation (CV), we used the *Relative Expression Variability* (REV). REV is the Bonferroni-like corrected mid-interval of the chi-square estimate of the pooled CV for all quantifiable transcripts of the same gene [17]

$$REV_i^{(NOR/PTC)} = \frac{1}{2}\underbrace{\left(\sqrt{\frac{r_i}{\chi^2(r_i;0.975)}} + \sqrt{\frac{r_i}{\chi^2(r_i;0.025)}}\right)}_{\text{correction coefficient}} \underbrace{\sqrt{\frac{1}{R_i}\sum_{k=1}^{R_i}\left(\frac{s_{ik}^{(NOR/PTC)}}{\mu_{ik}^{(NOR/PTC)}}\right)^2}}_{\text{pooled CV}} \times 100\% \quad (2)$$

μ_{ik} = average expression level of gene i probed by spot k (= 1, ..., R_i) in the 4 biological replicas
s_{ik} = standard deviation of the expression level of gene i probed by spot k
$r_i = 4R_i - 1$ = number of degrees of freedom
R_i = number of microarray spots probing redundantly gene i

A lower *REV* indicates stronger control by the cellular homeostatic mechanisms to limit the expression fluctuations, expected for genes critical for survival, proliferation and phenotypic expression. Therefore, we also use the *Relative Expression Control* (REC)

$$REC_i^{(NOR,PTC)} \equiv \frac{\langle REV \rangle^{(NOR/PTC)}}{REV_i^{(NOR/PTC)}} - 1 \quad (3)$$

$\langle \rangle$ = median for all genes profiled in that phenotype

As defined, positive *RECs* point to genes that are more controlled than the median while negative *RECs* identify less controlled genes in that phenotype. It is natural to assume that the cell invests more energy to control the expressions of more important genes for its survival, phenotypic expression and integration into a multi-cellular structure. As such, *REC* is a major factor to consider in establishing the gene hierarchy.

2.2.3. Expression Coordination

The expression coordination of two genes in the same region was quantified by their pair-wise momentum-product Pearson correlation coefficient between the two sets of expression levels across biological replicas, "$\rho_{ij}^{(NOR/PTC)}$". The statistical significance was evaluated with the two-tail t-test for the degrees of freedom df = 4(biological replicas)*R (number of spots probing redundantly each of the correlated transcripts) − 2. Two genes were considered as synergistically expressed (positive or in-phase coordination) if their expression levels fluctuated in phase across biological replicas. They are considered as antagonistically expressed (negative or anti-phase coordination) when their expression levels manifest opposite tendencies and are independently expressed (neutral coordination) when the expression fluctuations of one gene are not related to the fluctuations of the other [17]. Although not (yet) validated through molecular biology studies, the expression coordination was speculated to reflect the "transcriptomic stoichiometry" of the encoded proteins that are produced in certain proportions to optimize the cellular functional pathways [18].

We also computed the coordination power $CP_{i,\Gamma}^{(NOR/PTC)}$ [19] and the Overall Coordination $OC_{i,\Gamma}^{(NOR/PTC)}$ of a gene "i" with respect to the functional pathway "Γ" in each of the two profiled regions (NOR and PTC)

$$CP_{i,\Gamma}^{(NOR/PTC)} \equiv \overline{\rho_{ij}^{(NOR/PTC)}}\Big|_{\forall j \in \Gamma, j \neq i} \times 100\%, \quad OC_{i,\Gamma}^{(NOR/PTC)} \equiv \exp\left(\frac{4}{N}\sum_{j \in \Gamma, j \neq i} \rho_{ij}^2 - 1\right) \quad (4)$$

Both $CP_{i,\Gamma}^{(NOR/PTC)}$ and $OC_{i,\Gamma}^{(NOR/PTC)}$ are measures of the gene "i" influence on "Γ".

2.3. Gene Commanding Height (GCH) and Gene Master Regulator (GMR)

In previous papers [8–10], we introduced the Gene Commanding Height (GCH), a combination of the expression control and expression coordination with all (ALL) other genes, to establish the gene hierarchy in each phenotype

$$GCH_i^{(NOR,PTC)} \equiv \left(REC_i^{(NOR,PTC)} + 1\right)OC_{i,ALL}^{(NOR/PTC)} \equiv \frac{\langle REV \rangle^{(NOR/PTC)}}{REV_i^{(NOR/PTC)}} \exp\left(\frac{4}{N}\sum_{j \in ALL, j \neq i} \rho_{ij}^2 - 1\right) \quad (5)$$

The top gene (highest GCH) in each phenotype was termed Gene Master Regulator (GMR) of that phenotype. The very strict control of the GMR expression suggests that this gene is utterly important for cell survival, while the very high overall coordination indicates how much its expression regulates the expression of many other genes.

2.4. Expression Regulation

A gene was considered as significantly regulated in the PTC with respect to the NOR if the absolute expression ratio exceeds the cut-off (CUT) value computed individually for each gene by considering the expression variabilities of that gene in both compared conditions [9].

$$\left|x_i^{(NOR \rightarrow PTC)}\right| > CUT_i = 1 + \frac{1}{100}\sqrt{2\left(\left(REV_i^{(NOR)}\right)^2 + \left(REV_i^{(PTC)}\right)^2\right)}, \quad \text{where:} \quad (6)$$

$$x_i \equiv \begin{cases} \frac{\mu_i^{(PTC)}}{\mu_i^{(NOR)}}, & \text{if } \mu_i^{(PTC)} > \mu_i^{(NOR)} \\ -\frac{\mu_i^{(NOR)}}{\mu_i^{(PTC)}}, & \text{if } \mu_i^{(PTC)} < \mu_i^{(NOR)} \end{cases}, \quad \mu_i^{(PTC/NOR)} = \frac{1}{R_i}\sum_{k=1}^{R_i} \mu_{ik}^{(PTC/NOR)}$$

The "CUT" criterion for individual genes eliminates the false positives and the false negatives selected by considering uniform absolute fold-change cut-off (e.g., 1.5x). In addition to the percentage of up- and down-regulated genes (that considers all genes as equal contributors to the alteration of a pathway), or the expression ratios "x", we prefer the Weighted Individual (gene) Regulation [20], "WIR":

$$WIR_i^{(NOR \rightarrow PTC)} \equiv \mu_i^{(NOR)} \frac{x_i}{|x_i|}(|x_i| - 1)(1 - p_i) \quad \text{where:}$$
$$\mu_i^{(NOR)} = \text{average expression in the normal tissue,} \quad (7)$$
$$p_i = \text{p-value of the regulation}$$

Note that in Equation (7), WIR takes into account the normal expression of that gene (i.e., in NOR), its expression ratio (PTC vs. NOR) and the confidence interval (1-p) of the regulation.

2.5. Quantifiers of the Functional Genomic Fabrics

The Kyoto Encyclopedia of Genes and Genomes [21,22] was used to select the genes involved in the thyroid hormone synthesis (THS), cell cycle (CC) and oxidative phosphorylation (OPH), as well as how experimental manipulation of the PTC GMR might regulate the programmed cell death (apoptosis, APO). Although almost all functional pathways were perturbed in cancer, THS, CC, OPH and APO were selected because of their importance for the thyroid function and cancer development. There are reports of altered THS in cancer progression and apoptosis (e.g., [23]) and the role of the thyroid hormone in regulating the cell-cycle [24] and the oxidative phosphorylation [25].

Median REC over a gene selection (e.g., apoptosis pathway) was used to compare the expression controls of that selection in different regions or two different gene selections in the same region. Alteration of the genomic fabrics was quantified by the average "X" of the absolute expression ratios and by Weighted Pathway Regulation (WPR), the average of the absolute *WIRs* over a particular "selection" of genes

$$X^{(NOR \to PTC)}_{selection} \equiv \overline{\left| x_i^{(NOR \to PTC)} \right|}_{\forall i \in selection}$$
$$WPR^{(NOR \to PTC)}_{selection} \equiv \overline{\left| WIR_i^{(NOR \to PTC)} \right|}_{\forall i \in selection} \quad (8)$$

3. Results

3.1. Overall Results

A total of 14,903 well-quantified unigenes in all PTC and NOR samples, and in BCPAP and 8505C cells before and after transfection with one of the four targeted genes, were considered in the sequent analyses. The groups redundantly probing the same transcript were replaced by their averages in each biological replica. Eukaryotic translation elongation factor 1 α 1 (*EEF1A1*) had the largest expression (82.31 median gene expression units) in NOR (not significantly regulated in PTC). Niemann-Pick disease, type C2 (*NPC2*) had the largest expression in PTC (86.97 median gene expression units), up-regulated by 7.24x with respect to NOR. Notch 1 (*NOTCH1*) with 82.35 had the largest expression in the BCPAP cells and myelin protein zero-like 3 (*MPZL3*) with 107.60 tops the gene expression level in the 8505C cells.

Out of the quantified unigenes, 1225 (8.22%) were down-regulated and 1852 (12.42%) were up-regulated in PTC with respect to NOR. The average absolute PTC/NOR expression ratio for all genes was $X = 1.768$ (median $|x| = 1.309$) and the *WPR* was 1.071 (median WIR = 0.046). Chitinase 3-like 1 (*CHI3L1*) was the most up-regulated ($x = 219.38$) and trefoil factor 3 (intestinal) (*TFF3*) the most down-regulated (x-99.86) gene in PTC. Because expression coordination and average expression level are independent measures, the high regulation of these genes in PTC with respect to NOR has no relevance for their networking in either of the two profiled regions.

3.2. Three Independent Measures for Each Gene

Figure 1 illustrates the independence of the three measures for the first 50 alphabetically ordered genes involved in the KEGG-derived [22] human apoptosis pathway (hsa04210). We chose *IL6* (interleukin 6) to illustrate the expression coordination of apoptotic genes owing to the significant role of the encoded protein (IL6) in the PTC development [26]. However, coordination with any other gene supports the same conclusion. In addition to the clear independence of the three measures, transcriptomic differences between the two histo-pathologically distinct profiled regions from the thyroid are evident.

In this gene selection, FBJ murine osteosarcoma viral oncogene homolog (*FOS*) has the highest average expression level (45.37) in NOR (significantly down-regulated by −2.06x in PTC). Cathepsin H (*CTSH*) had the largest expression (35.23), up-regulated by 6.78x with respect to NOR. *FOS*, cathepsin K (*CTSK*) and inhibitor of kappa light polypeptide gene enhancer in B-cells kinase γ (*IKBKG*) were among the significantly down-regulated genes. In contrast, *BID* (H3 interacting domain death agonist), *CTSH* and *DIABLO* (diablo, IAP-binding mitochondrial protein), were among the up-regulated genes of the selection.

CASP8 and FADD-like apoptosis regulator (*CLFAR*) was the most variably expressed gene in the normal tissue and DNA fragmentation factor (*DFFB*), 40kDa, β polypeptide (caspase-activated DNase) the most variably expressed in PTC. Note that most of the selected genes have larger expression variability in the normal tissue than in the cancer nodule. This result confirms our previous reports (see Discussions) about diseases triggering increased control exerted by the cellular homeostatic mechanisms on the transcripts abundances as a way to protect against extensive damages.

Observe also that 20 (40%) of the illustrated apoptotic genes are synergistically expressed with *IL6* in the normal tissue and only two (4%) in the PTC nodule, suggesting the decoupling of the programmed cell death from the inflammatory response in cancer.

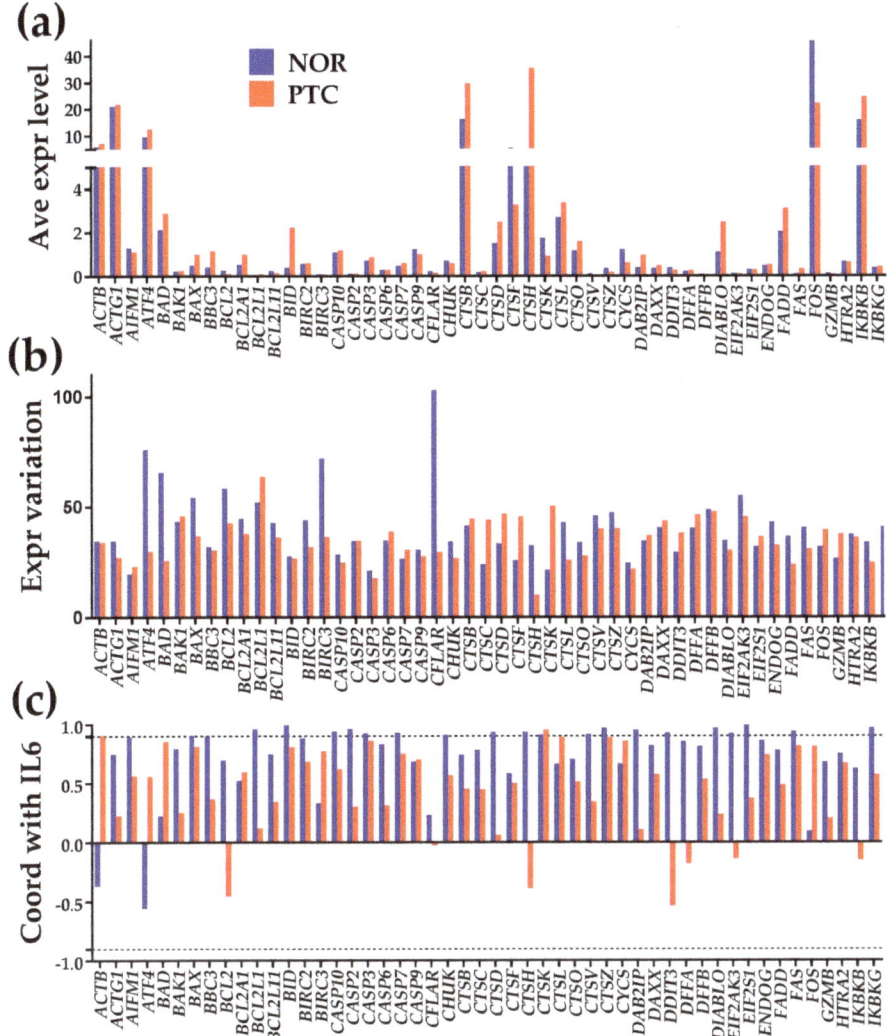

Figure 1. Three independent characteristics of every gene in each region. (**a**) average expression level, (**b**) expression variation and (**c**) expression coordination (here with IL6). The dashed black lines in panel (**c**) indicate the interval out of which the positive/negative coordination is considered as statistically significant.

3.3. Expression Regulation

Figure 2 illustrates the contributions of the first 50 alphabetically ordered quantified oncogenes to the overall regulation in PTC measured by the percentages of the up- and down-regulated genes, expression ratios and weighted individual (gene) regulations. The percentages are restricted to only the significantly regulated genes (considered as equal −1/+1 contributors). By contrast, both X and WIR take into account all (regulated and not regulated) genes and the contributions of these genes are no longer uniform. More informative than the expression ratio, WIR weights the contribution of each gene by its normal expression level (i.e., in NOR), fold-change in cancer and statistical significance of the regulation.

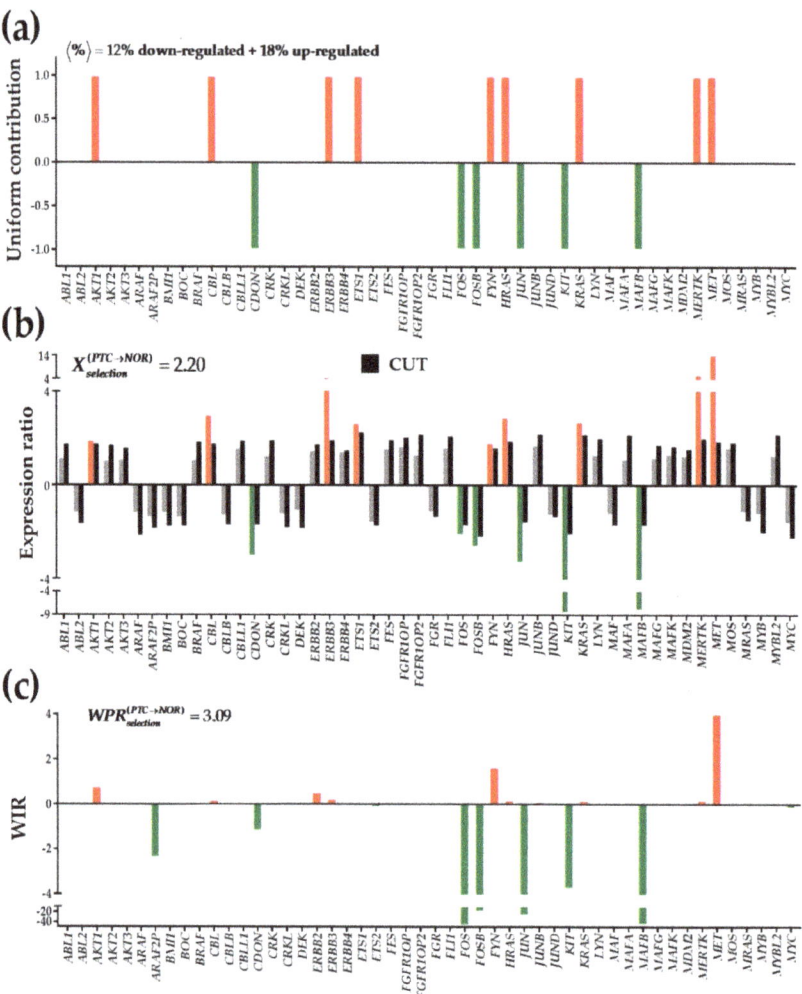

Figure 2. Three ways to consider the contribution of a gene to the pathway regulation. (**a**) uniform; (**b**) by expression ratio; (**c**) as Weighted Individual (gene) Regulation. Red/green/grey columns indicate up-/down-/not regulated genes. Black columns are the fold-change cut-offs (negative for down-regulation). Regulated genes: v-akt murine thymoma viral oncogene homolog 1 (*AKT1*), Cbl proto-oncogene, E3 ubiquitin protein ligase (*CBL*), cell adhesion associated, oncogene regulated (*CDON*), v-erb-b2 avian erythroblastic leukemia viral oncogene homolog 3 (*ERBB3*), v-ets avian erythroblastosis virus E26 oncogene homolog 1 (*ETS1*), homologs of FBJ murine osteosarcoma viral oncogene (*FOS/FOSB*), FYN proto-oncogene, Src family tyrosine kinase (*FYN*), Harvey rat sarcoma viral oncogene homolog (*HRAS*), jun proto-oncogene (*JUN*), Kirsten rat sarcoma viral oncogene homolog (*KRAS*), v-yes-1 Yamaguchi sarcoma viral related oncogene homolog (*LYN*), v-maf avian musculoaponeurotic fibrosarcoma oncogene homolog B (*MAFB*), c-mer proto-oncogene tyrosine kinase (*MERTK*) and met proto-oncogene (*MET*).

3.4. Regulation of the Thyroid Hormone Synthesis

Figure 3 presents the regulations of the genes involved in the (KEGG-determined) thyroid hormone synthesis (hsa04918). In this pathway, 10.0 (20%) of the 50 quantified genes were up-regulated and six (12%) were down-regulated.

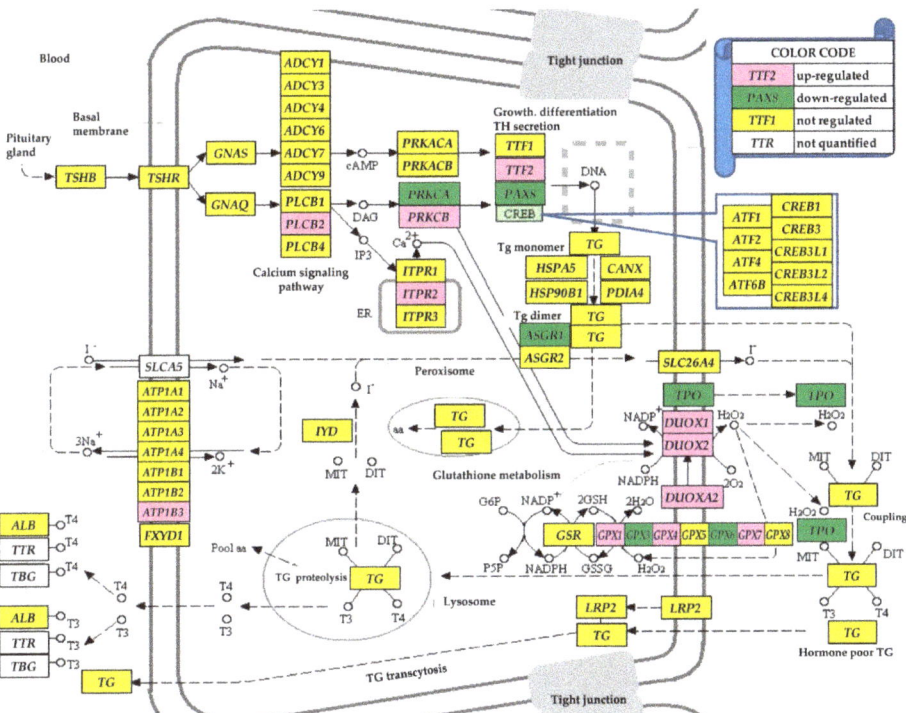

Figure 3. Regulation of thyroid hormone synthesis pathway (modified from hsa04918). Regulated genes: asialoglycoprotein receptor 1 (*ASGR1*), ATPase, Na+/K+ transporting, β 3 polypeptide (*ATP1B3*), dual oxidases (*DUOX1/2*), dual oxidase maturation factor 2 (*DUOXA2*), glutathione peroxidases (*GPX1/3/4/6/7*), inositol 1,4,5-trisphosphate receptor, type 2 (*ITPR2*), paired box 8 (*PAX8*), protein kinases C (*PRKCA/B*), thyroid peroxidase (*TPO*) and transcription termination factor, RNA polymerase II (*TTF2*).

3.5. Regulation of the Cell-Cycle Pathway

Figure 4 presents the regulation of the genes involved in the (KEGG-determined) cell cycle pathway (hsa04110), where, out of the 93 genes quantified, three (3.23%) were down-regulated and 14 (15.05%) were up-regulated. Except *PTTG2*, all other regulated genes are located in the DNA replication (S-phase) and the two temporal gaps, G1 and G2, separating the S phase from mitosis (M-phase), indicating faster replication but stationary differentiation.

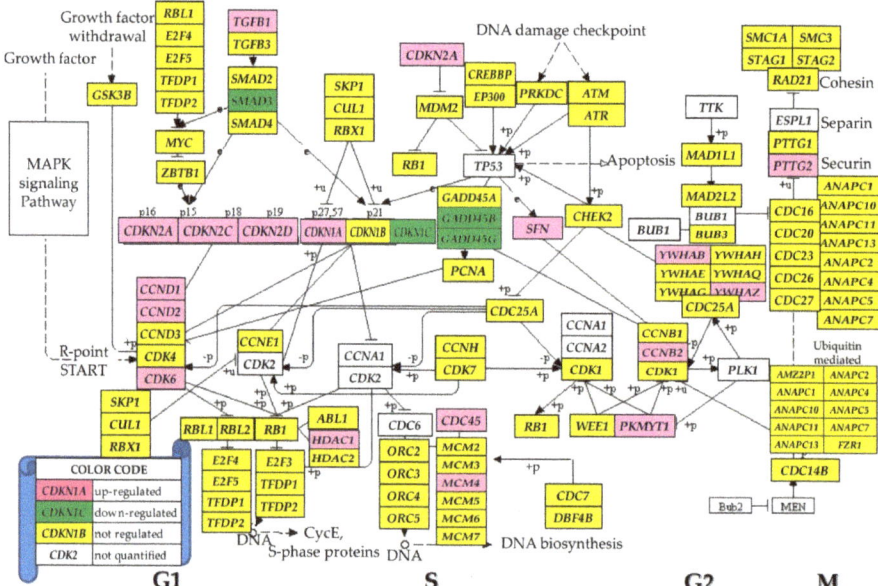

Figure 4. Regulation of the KEGG-determined cell cycle (hsa04110). Regulated genes: cyclins (*CCNB2/D1/D2*), cell division cycle 45 (*CDC45*), cyclin-dependent kinase inhibitors (*CDKN1A/1C/2A/2C/2D*), growth arrest and DNA-damage-inducibles (*GADD45B/D*), histone deacetylase 1 (*HDAC1*), minichromosome maintenance complex component 4 (*MCM4*), membrane associated tyrosine/threonine 1 (*PKMYT1*), pituitary tumor-transforming 2 (*PTTG2*), stratifin (*SFN*), SMAD family member 3 (*SMAD3*), transforming growth factor, β 1 (*TGFB1*) and tyrosine 3-monooxygenase/tryptophan 5-monooxygenase activation proteins (*YWHAB/Z*).

3.6. Remodeling of the Oxidative Phosphorylation Pathway

Figure 5 presents the remodeling of the coordination networks interlinking the five complexes ([C1], [C2], [C3], [C4], [C5]) of the oxidative phosphorylation in the PTC nodule with respect to NOR tissue. The genes were selected from the KEGG hsa 00190. Note the substantial increase in the synergistically expressed gene pairs in PTC (273) with respect of the NOR (155) and that there is no antagonistically expressed gene pair in PTC, while in NOR there are 105. When the coordination inside each complex is added, there are 781 synergistic and 0 antagonistic pairs in PTC versus 458 synergistic and 242 antagonistic pairs in NOR. In addition to the eight up-regulated and three down-regulated genes within the selection of the 92 oxidative-phosphorylation genes, these results indicate a significant increase in the coordination of the complexes involved in the OP activity.

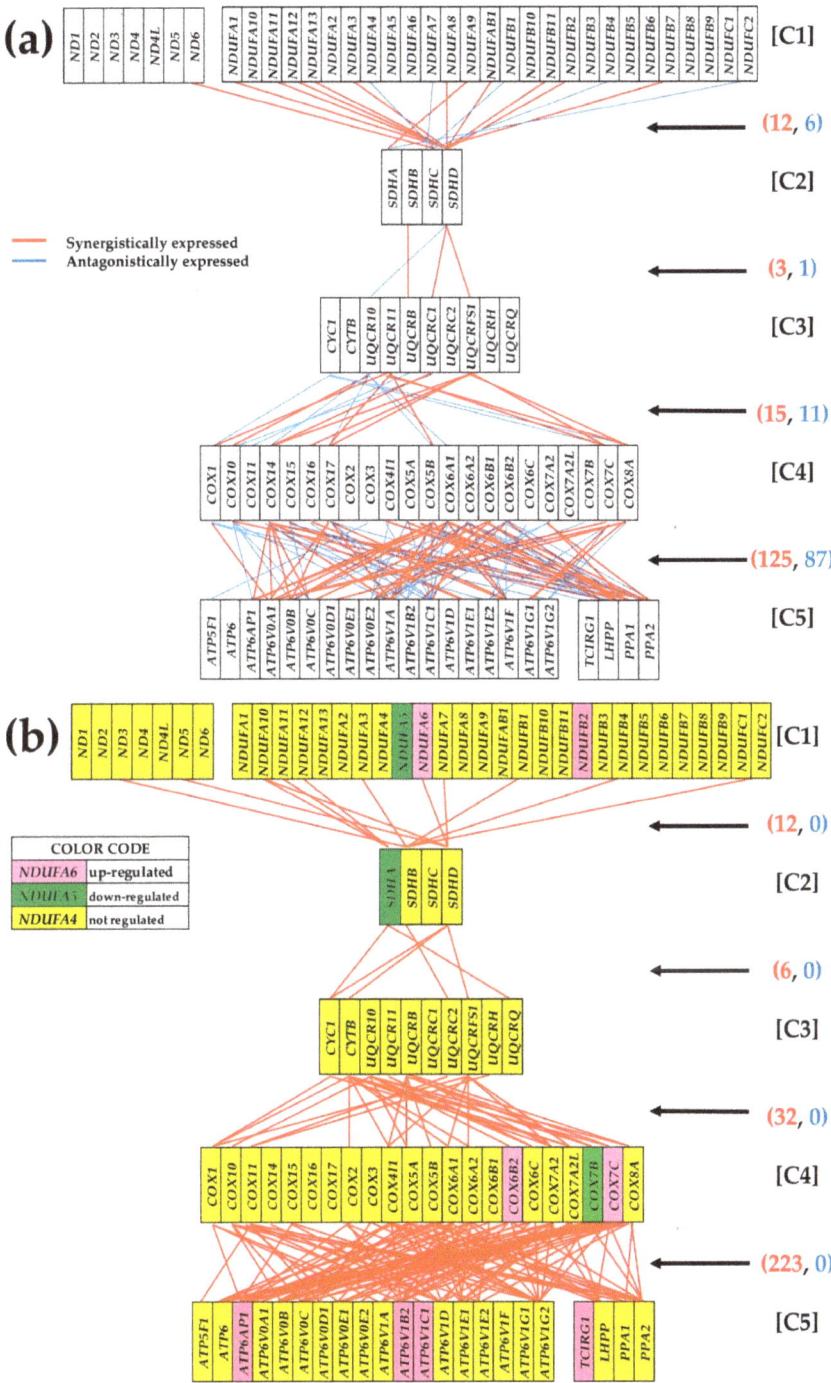

Figure 5. Remodeling of the coordination networks among the five complexes of the oxidative phosphorylation in the PTC nodule with respect to NOR tissue. The red/blue lines indicate that the

connected genes are synergistically/antagonistically expressed in that region. Red/blue numbers in parentheses indicate the number of synergistically/antagonistically expressed gene pairs between the two complexes. Regulated genes: ATPase, H+ transporting, lysosomal proteins (*ATP6AP1*, *ATP6V1B2*, *ATP6V1C1*), cytochrome c oxidase subunits (*COX6B2*, *COX7B*, *COX7C*), NADH dehydrogenase (ubiquinone) 1 α/β subcomplexes (*NDUFA5*, *NDUFA6*, *NDUFB2*), succinate dehydrogenase complex, subunit A, flavoprotein (Fp) (*SDHA*) and T-cell, immune regulator 1, ATPase, H+ transporting, lysosomal V0 subunit A3 (*TCIRG1*).

3.7. Gene Hierarchy

Figure 6 presents the GCH scores of the 12 most frequently mutated genes in TC (reported in [1]) and the top 12 genes in NOR and PTC. Mutated genes: B double prime 1, subunit of RNA polymerase III transcription initiation factor IIIB (*BDP1*), B-Raf proto-oncogene, serine/threonine kinase (*BRAF*), *DST* (dystonin), eukaryotic translation initiation factor 1A, X-linked (*EIF1AX*), Harvey rat sarcoma viral oncogene homolog (*HRAS*), lysine (K)-specific methyltransferase 2A (*KMT2A*), microtubule-actin crosslinking factor 1 (*MACR1*), metastasis associated lung adenocarcinoma transcript 1 (non-protein coding) (*MALAT1*), neuroblastoma RAS viral (v-ras) oncogene homolog (*NRAS*), thyroglobulin (*TG*), ubiquitin-specific peptidase 9, X-linked (*USP9X*), zinc finger homeobox 3 (*ZFHX3*). Note that none of the most frequently mutated genes are among the top 12 genes in either region. Even *BRAF*, mutated in 20.56% of the 1440 cases, has no competitive GCH to be a good candidate for the PTC gene therapy (GCH of *BRAF* in PTC is 11.79). However, *SPINT2*, the PTC's GMR ($GCH_{SPINT2}^{(PTC)}$ = 54.97), appears to be the most legitimate target for this case. While significant alteration of the expression of *SPINT2* would have lethal impact on the cancer cells, due to the very low GCH in NOR ($GCH_{SPINT2}^{(NOR)}$ = 1.93), it might have very little consequences on the normal cells. Importantly, the GCH scores of the top genes in PTC are substantially lower in NOR and vice-versa.

For comparison, we added the GCH scores of the top 23 genes in each of the standard TC cell lines BCPAP (papillary) and 8505C (anaplastic). Remarkably, 14 genes in the BCPAP cells and three genes in the 8505C cells have GCH scores higher than *SPINT2* in PTC. As an additional reference, Figure S1 shows the GCH scores of most of the genes from FoundationOne®CDx (Foundation Medicine, Cambridge, MA, U.S.A.) used by Foundation Medicine [7] for genomic testing of solid tumors, including "Non-Small Cell Lung (NSCLC), Colorectal, Breast, Ovarian, and Melanoma. The list contains genes with full coding exonic regions for the detection of substitutions, insertion-deletions (indels), and copy-number alterations (CNAs). It also includes genes with select intronic regions for the detection of gene rearrangements, one gene with a promoter region (telomerase reverse transcriptase (*TERT*)) and one non-coding RNA gene (*TERC*). These genes might be useful for diagnostic purposes. However, with their GCH score far below the GMR's and with not enough difference between PTC and NOR, they should have little therapeutic value for this particular case. Substantially lower than the PTC GMR were the biomarkers, oncogenes, apoptosis genes and the ncRNAs determined in the same specimens and presented in Figure 2 from [8].

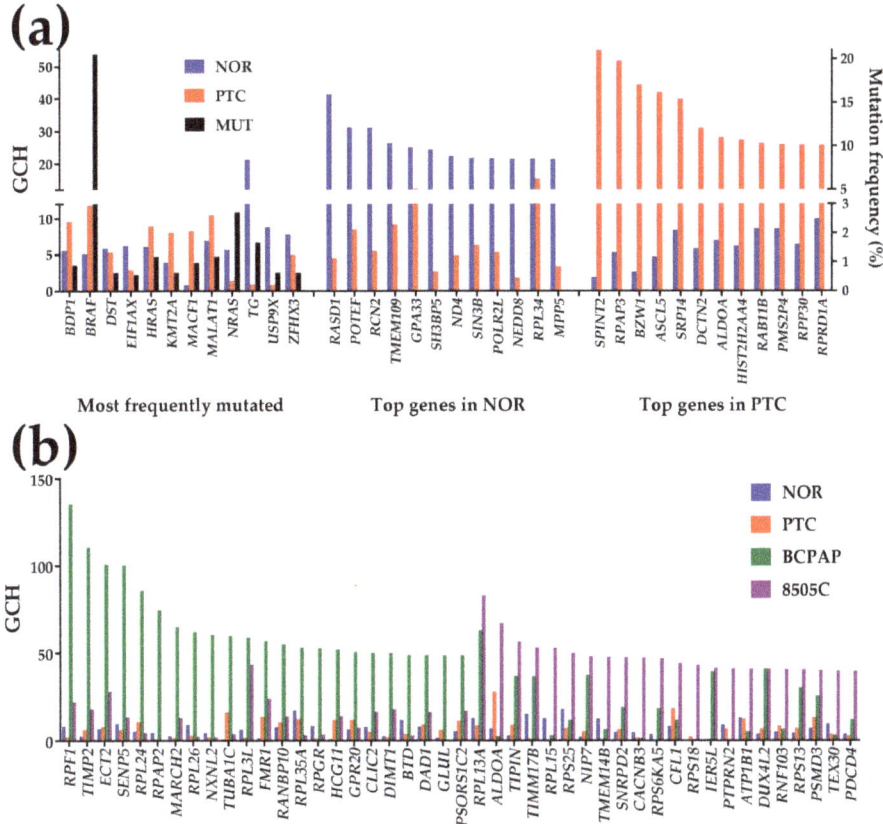

Figure 6. Gene Commanding Height (GCH). (**a**) GCH and mutation frequency of the 12 reported most frequently mutated genes and the top 12 genes in the normal tissue (NOR) and the papillary nodule (PTC). The mutation frequency is plotted on the right axis. (**b**) GCH of the top 23 genes in the papillary (BCPAP) and anaplastic (8505C) thyroid cancer cell lines and their scores in NOR and PTC. Top 3 genes in NOR: RAS, dexamethasone-induced 1 (*RASD1*), POTE ankyrin domain family, member F (*POTEF*), reticulocalbin 2, EF-hand calcium binding domain (*RCN2*). Top 3 genes in PTC: serine peptidase inhibitor, Kunitz type, 2 (*SPINT2*), RNA polymerase II associated protein 3 (*RPAP3*), basic leucine zipper and W2 domains 1 (*BZW1*). Top 3 genes in BCPAP cells: ribosome production factor 1 homolog (S. cerevisiae) (*RPF1*), TIMP metallopeptidase inhibitor 2 (*TIMP2*), epithelial cell transforming 2 (*ECT2*). Top 3 genes in 8505C cells: ribosomal protein L13a (*RPL13A*), aldolase A, fructose-bisphosphate (*ALDOA*), TIMELESS interacting protein (*TIPIN*).

3.8. The Gene Master Regulator at Play

Our study identified *SPINT2*, a not regulated gene in the investigated PTA, as the GMR of this patient's malignancy. What are the mechanisms by which experimental alteration of *SPINT2* expression might selectively kill the cancer cells but not the normal ones? *SPINT2* is highly coordinated with numerous genes from almost all major functional pathways. However, we considered that apoptosis might be the best candidate to evaluate (from a bioinformatics point of view) the effects of *SPINT2* manipulation. Therefore, we analyzed the expression coordination of *SPINT2* with the 112 apoptosis genes quantified in the two regions. Table 1 presents the apoptosis genes that are significantly up/down regulated in PTC or/and significantly synergistically/antagonistically/independently expressed with *SPINT2* in NOR or/and PTC.

Table 1. Apoptosis genes that are significantly up(U)/down(D) regulated in PTC with respect to NOR or/and significantly synergistically (S)/antagonistically (A)/independently (I) expressed with *SPINT2* in NOR or/and PTC.

GENE	DESCRIPTION	NOR	PTC	REG
ACTG1	actin, γ 1	S		
AKT1	v-akt murine thymoma viral oncogene homolog 1			U
AKT3	v-akt murine thymoma viral oncogene homolog 3		S	
ATF4	activating transcription factor 4	A		
ATM	ataxia telangiectasia mutated		S	
BAK1	BCL2-antagonist/killer 1		S	
BAX	BCL2-associated X protein			U
BBC3	BCL2 binding component 3		S	U
BCL2	B-cell CLL/lymphoma 2	I		
BCL2A1	BCL2-related protein A1			U
BCL2L1	BCL2-like 1		S	
BCL2L11	BCL2-like 11		S	
BID	BH3 interacting domain death agonist			U
BIRC5	baculoviral IAP repeat containing 5			U
CAPN1	calpain 1, (mu/I) large subunit		S	
CASP2	caspase 2, apoptosis-related cysteine peptidase		S	
CASP3	caspase 3, apoptosis-related cysteine peptidase			U
CASP6	caspase 6, apoptosis-related cysteine peptidase		S	
CASP9	caspase 9, apoptosis-related cysteine peptidase	S		
CFLAR	CASP8 and FADD-like apoptosis regulator		S	
CTSC	cathepsin C			U
CTSD	cathepsin D		S	
CTSH	cathepsin H			U
CTSK	cathepsin K			D
CTSL	cathepsin L	S		
CTSV	cathepsin V		S	
CYCS	cytochrome c, somatic	S		D
DAB2IP	DAB2 interacting protein		S	U
DFFA	DNA fragmentation factor		S	
DIABLO	diablo, IAP-binding mitochondrial protein		S	U
EIF2AK3	eukaryotic translation initiation factor 2-α kinase 3		S	
EIF2S1	eukaryotic translation initiation factor 2, subunit 1 α		S	
FAS	Fas cell surface death receptor			U
FOS	FBJ murine osteosarcoma viral oncogene homolog			D
GZMB	granzyme B (granzyme 2, cytotoxic T-lymphocyte-associated serine esterase 1)		S	D
IKBKB	inhibitor of kappa light polypeptide gene enhancer in B-cells, kinase β	I	S	
ITPR2	inositol 1,4,5-trisphosphate receptor, type 2			U
JUN	jun proto-oncogene			D
LMNA	lamin A/C			U
LMNB2	lamin B2		S	
MAP2K1	mitogen-activated protein kinase kinase 1			U
MAP2K2	mitogen-activated protein kinase kinase 2		S	
MAP3K9	mitogen-activated protein kinase kinase kinase 9		S	
MAPK1	mitogen-activated protein kinase 1		S	
MAPK3	mitogen-activated protein kinase 3		S	
NFKB1	nuclear factor of kappa light polypeptide gene enhancer in B-cells 1	S		
NFKBIA	nuclear factor of kappa light polypeptide gene enhancer in B-cells inhibitor, α			D
NRAS	neuroblastoma RAS viral (v-ras) oncogene homolog		S	
PARP1	poly (ADP-ribose) polymerase 1			U
PARP4	poly (ADP-ribose) polymerase family, member 4		S	
PDPK1	3-phosphoinositide dependent protein kinase 1		S	
PIK3CA	phosphatidylinositol-4,5-bisphosphate 3-kinase, catalytic subunit α		S	

Table 1. Cont.

GENE	DESCRIPTION	NOR	PTC	REG
PIK3R1	phosphoinositide-3-kinase, regulatory subunit 1			D
PIK3R2	phosphoinositide-3-kinase, regulatory subunit 2		S	U
PMAIP1	phorbol-12-myristate-13-acetate-induced protein 1		S	U
RAF1	v-raf-1 murine leukemia viral oncogene homolog 1	S		
RELA	v-rel avian reticuloendotheliosis viral oncogene homolog A		S	
TNFRSF10B	tumor necrosis factor receptor superfamily, member 10b			U
TNFRSF1A	tumor necrosis factor receptor superfamily, member 1A		S	U
TRAF2	TNF receptor-associated factor 2		S	
TUBA1C	tubulin, α 1b	I		
TUBA3D	tubulin, α 3c	I		
TUBA4A	tubulin, α 4a			U
XIAP	X-linked inhibitor of apoptosis		S	

In PTC (21 significantly up-regulated and seven down-regulated apoptosis genes), we found *SPINT2* to be significantly synergistically expressed with 34 apoptosis genes, but with no significant antagonistically or independently expressed partners. This is a substantial increase from the six synergistically, one antagonistically and four independently expressed apoptosis partners of *SPINT2* in NOR. Interestingly, none of the significant correlations in NOR (with: *ACTG1*, *ATF4*, *CASP9*, *CTSL*, *CYCS*, *NFKB1*) were maintained in PTC.

What effect the overexpression of an otherwise stably expressed but not regulated gene in PTC (*SPINT2*) may have on cancer cells? Most probably, owing to the substantial expression synergistic coordination with apoptosis genes, the experimental overexpression of *SPINT2* would up-regulate many of these genes, forcing the commanded (PTC) cells to enter programmed death.

There was no way to validate this hypothesis on the patient from whom we had profiled the thyroid tumor. However, we tested the general hypothesis that expression coordination with one gene predicts expression regulation when the expression of that gene is experimentally manipulated. For this purpose, we analyzed the transcriptomes of the TC cell lines BCPAP and 8505C cells before and after stable lentiviral transfection with either *DDX19B*, *NEMP1*, *PANK2* or *UBALD1* [8]. Figure 7a,b plots the correlation coefficient with *DDX19B* in the untreated cells against the fold-changes (negative for down-regulation) of the genes in the transfected cells. They clearly show that expression coordination predicts (>86%) the expression regulation with reasonable accuracy. Similar validation (83–91%) was obtained for the same cell lines transfected with either *NEMP1*, *PANK2* or *UBALD1*. Based on this validation, Figure 7c illustrates the predicted regulations of apoptosis genes if the expression level of *SPINT2* in PTC is significantly increased.

In Figure 7c, we used the uniform contribution of the significantly altered genes to the percentages of (up-/down-) regulated genes. Note that from 21 up-regulated and six down-regulated genes in untreated PTC, overexpression of *SPINT2* may result in 48 up-regulated and six down-regulated genes. The expression of six genes, *BBC3*, *DAB2IP*, *DIABLO*, *PIK3R2*, *PMAIP1*, *TNFRSF1A*, which are already up-regulated in PTC may be further increased by treatment, while the down-regulation of *GZMB* in untreated PTC may be recovered by overexpressing *SINT2*.

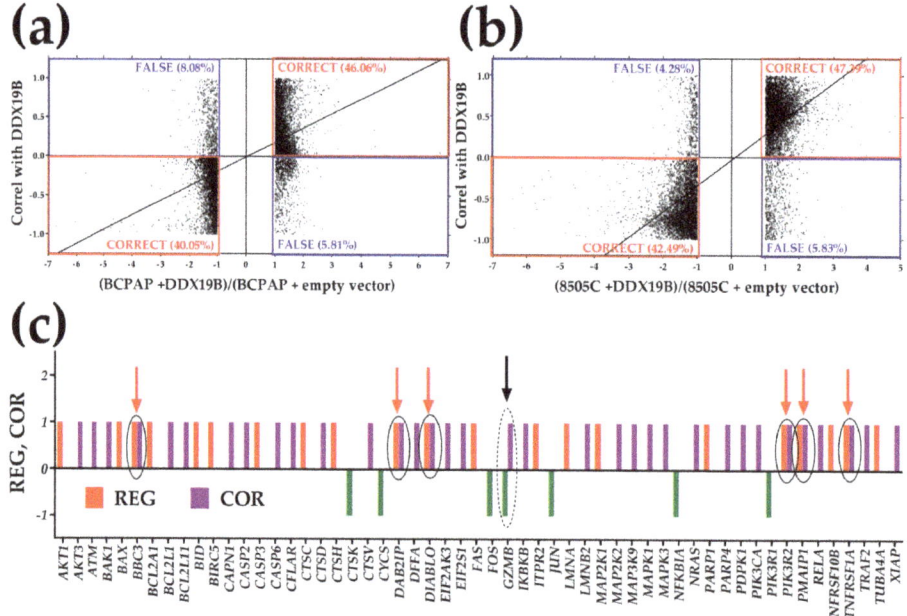

Figure 7. Prediction of the ripple effects of experimental gene regulation. (**a**) Expression coordination with *DDX19B* in untreated BCAP cells accurately predicts 86.11% (40.05 + 46.06) the type of the expression regulation in BCAP cells stably transfected with *DDX19B*; (**b**) Expression coordination with *DDX19B* in untreated 8505C cells accurately predicts 89.88% (42.49 + 47.39) of the type of the expression regulation in 8505C cells stably transfected with *DDX19B*; (**c**) Predicted regulation (1 for up-regulation and −1 for down-regulation) of apoptotic genes in PTC following experimental overexpression of *SPINT2*. REG = significant (1 = up-regulation, −1 = down-regulation). COR = significant expression synergism. Only the regulated genes in the untreated PTC and those expected to be regulated in treated PTC are represented. Red arrows indicate combined effect in treated tumor of regulation and expression synergism in untreated PTC. The black arrow indicates the down-regulation in untreated PTC expected to be compensated by the overexpression of *SPINT2*.

4. Discussion

Although with no molecular biology validation, the bioinformatics analysis of the gene expression profiles in the cancer nodule and surrounding normal tissue of a surgically removed papillary tumor produced some very interesting results, out of which the most important are:

1. Each cell phenotype from the tumor is governed by a different gene hierarchy and a distinct organization of its transcriptome;
2. As selected from the most altered genes in a large population of cancer patients, the biomarkers have low GCH and therefore little therapeutic value;
3. The GMR of the cancer nodule is the most legitimate target of the gene therapy because it is the most influential gene for cancer cells while having very little role in the surrounding normal cells;
4. *SPINT2* was identified as the GMR of the PTC nodule of the profiled tumor and a gene with very low GCH score in NOR;
5. The up-regulation of the synergistically expressed apoptosis genes in untreated PTC following the experimental *SPINT2* overexpression was identified as a potential mechanism of selectively killing the cancer cells.

The analysis presented in this report is consistent with the genomic fabric paradigm [11] that considers the transcriptome as a multi-dimensional object subjected to a dynamic set of expression correlations among the genes. The traditional transcriptomic analysis is limited to the expression level of individual genes and comparisons of the expression levels of distinct genes in the same condition or of the same gene in different conditions. Our procedure considerably enlarges the transcriptomic information by considering for each gene not one, but three independent features and all possible combinations of these features to compare the genes and groups of genes in the same condition or across various conditions.

Although high levels of *EEF1A1* were reported in renal cell carcinoma [27], we found this gene to have the highest expression in NOR and one of the highest levels in PTC (68.47), albeit not significantly down-regulated. A high expression of *NPC2* and its significant elevation in PTC were also detected in meta-analyses of public PTC transcriptomes [28]. Overexpression of *CHI3L1*, the most up-regulated gene in the analyzed PTC, was reported as associated with metastatic PTC [29] and its recurrence [30]. Significantly decreased expression of *TFF3*, the most down-regulated gene in our study, was also reported in several other studies (e.g., [31]).

In addition to illustrating the independence of the three features, Figure 1 provides also some interesting findings and confirmations of results reported by other authors. For instance, the high expression of *CTSH* in PTC (up-regulated by 6.78x with respect to NOR) was related to the tumor progression and migration of cancer cells [32].

The median REV has a statistically significant (p-value = 7.79×10^{-5}) decrease from 39.75 in NOR to 38.69 in PTC. According to the Second Law of Thermodynamics, the significantly larger overall expression variability in NOR than in PTC indicates not only relaxed control by the homeostatic mechanisms (average REC_{NOR} = 0.084, average REC_{PTC} = 0.113), but also that NOR is closer to the thermodynamic (here physiological) equilibrium. Supporting this assertion is the reduction in the median REV observed by us in all other gene expression studies on animal models of human diseases (e.g., [33–35]) and in tissues of animals subjected to various stresses (e.g., [36–38] or to genetic manipulations (e.g., [39,40]). The high expression variability of *CFLAR* (a key anti-apoptosis regulator [41]) in NOR (REV = 102.93) may explain the adaptability of the apoptosis pathway to a large spectrum of environmental conditions. The *CFLAR* REV dramatic reduction in PTC (REV = 29.41) shows the need for tighter control of resisting apoptosis in cancer. Moreover, its reduction in expression level (in PTC by −1.64x) was associated with delayed apoptosis [41].

The observed down-regulation of *FOS* in PTC (Figure 2) confirms the findings of some groups [42,43] but contradicts its frequent (however not 100%) up-regulation reported by another group in 40 patients with thyroid cancer and 20 with benign thyroid diseases [44]. Let us analyze what measure of regulation is the most informative and use the examples of *FOS* and *KIT* (another gene down-regulated in thyroid cancer [45]). Although both genes account as units for the percentage of the down-regulated genes, they contribute −2.06x and −8.15x as expression ratios and −46.28 and −3.76 as WIRs. Since WIR is a more comprehensive measure, *FOS* regulation appears to be the most important factor in the alteration of this group of genes. Indeed, FOS protein is an important player in cell proliferation, differentiation, transformation and apoptotic cell death.

Among the significantly regulated genes from the KEGG-derived THS pathway (Figure 3), only *PAX8* (−1.94x) was previously related to the thyroid cancer, albeit to the follicular form. Moreover, we found that peroxisome proliferator-activated receptor γ (*PPARG*) whose fusion with *PAX8* is considered an important trigger of the FTC [46], was likewise significantly down-regulated (−4.99x). Interestingly, in Figure 3, the two glutathione peroxidases, *GPX1* (1.60x) and *GPX3* (−1.84x), were oppositely regulated. Since the down-regulation of *GPX1* was reported to augment the pro-inflammatory cytokine-induced redox signaling and endothelial cell activation [47], one may assume that up-regulation of *GPX1* will do the opposite, i.e., diminish the pro-inflammatory cytokine-induced redox signaling. As such, the PTC cells will become more resistant to the inflammatory response.

According to the KEGG map hsa04110, some of the regulated cell-cycle genes (Figure 4) were associated with a wide diversity of cancers. Thus, up-regulation of *CDKN1A* was associated with cervical cancer [48] and down-regulation of *CDKN1C* with gastric cancer [49]. As stated in [3], up-regulation/mutation of *CDKN2A* was detected in numerous cancer forms: neoplasms (squamous cell, ductal, lobular, cystic, mucinous, serous, mesothelial, lipomathous, myomathous, thymic epithelial, complex, mixed), adenomas, adenocarcionmas, gliomas, nevi and melanomas, transitional cell papillomas and carcinomas, mature B-cell lymphomas, soft tissue tumors and sarcomas. *CDKN2B* was associated with malignant pleural mesothelioma, osteosarcoma and meningioma. However, we found no report associating these genes with thyroid cancer. Unfortunately, one of the most cancer-related genes, *TP53* [50], was not quantified in this experiment due to the corrupted probing spot in one of the microarrays, which can be seen as a major limitation of the study.

As illustrated in Figure 5 for interlinks between the five complexes of the oxidative phosphorylation, cancer remodels the gene networks, profoundly perturbing the mitochondrial function [51]. Among others, 10 synergistically expressed gene pairs in NOR are switched into antagonistically expressed pairs in PTC: *NDUFA10-SDHD, CYC1-COX1, COX10-ATP6V0B, COX10-ATP6V0C, COX5B-LHPP, COX6A1-ATV1B2, COX6A1-LHPP, COX6A2-ATP6V0B, COX6A2-ATP6V1A, COX7C-ATP6V1G2*. These switches, the cancellation of all significant antagonisms and the added synergisms increase the expression synchrony of the pathway genes [17] and remove the controlling bottlenecks. In a synergistic pair, the up-regulation of one gene triggers the up-regulation of the other. Although in this experiment we did not detect significantly altered expressions of *NDUFA10* and *SDHD*, their significant synergism in PTC may explain why they are both up-regulated in oral cancer [52].

Given the never-repeatable set of risk factors, each patient is unique and therefore their gene hierarchy is unique. Although the chance of finding the same GMR in two persons is about 1/20,000 and that of the first two genes is 1/400 million, from the first three genes up, the number of possibilities (7.9988×10^{12}) exceeds by far the Earth human population. Therefore, the top three genes are enough to uniquely represent the cancer of each person at a given time. In our studied PTC, the top three genes were: *SPINT2, RPAP3* and *BZW,1* with none of them significantly regulated with respect to NOR.

SPINT2, the identified GMR of the profiled PTC (Figure 6), was previously reported by several groups to be involved in the development and progression of a wide diversity of forms of cancer [53]. Among others, *SPINT2* was associated with metastatic osteosarcoma [54], ovarian cancer [55], glioma/glioblastoma [56,57], prostate cancer [58] and non-small lung cancer [59], leukemia [60] and cervical carcinoma [61]. *RPAP3*, essential for assembling chaperone complexes [62], was linked to hypoxia-adapted cancer cells [63] and *BZW,1* was associated with ovarian [64], lung [65] and salivary gland [66] cancers. However, we found no mention in the literature about the role of these first three genes in any form of thyroid cancer.

In Figure 7 and Table 1, we tested whether expression synergism with apoptosis genes may be one of the mechanisms by which manipulation of *SPINT2* expression is lethal to the PTC cells but not to the NOR cells. First, we determined the significant coordination of *SPINT2* with apoptosis genes in both NOR and PTC and found a substantial increase in the expression synergism in PTC. Then, we tested the predictive value of the expression coordination by profiling two standard human TC cell lines before and after stable transfection with four genes selected, only to have substantially different GCHs in the two cell lines. Although *DDX19B* and *PANK2* (but not *NEMP1* and *UBALD1*) were synergistically expressed with *SPINT2* in PTC, there are no reports relating these genes with *SPINT2* in any form of cancer. As mentioned in [8], *NEMP1* and *PANK2* had higher GCHs and induced larger transcriptomic alterations in the BCPAP than in the 8505C cells. In contrast, *DDX19B* and *UBALD1* had higher GCHs and induced larger transcriptomic alterations in the 8505C than in the BCPAP cells. Figure 7a,b confirms our previous findings that expression correlation with one gene predicts what genes are regulated when the expression of that gene is manipulated. A similar conclusion was drawn in [67], where we had shown that most genes are synergistically/antagonistically expressed with *Gja* (encoding the gap junction protein Cx43) in the brain and hearts of wildtype mice are down-/up-regulated in the brain and hearts of Cx43KO mice. Therefore, as illustrated in Figure 7c, we expect that, due to the synergism, the overexpression of *SPINT2* will force the PTC cells into programmed death by up-regulating numerous apoptosis genes.

5. Conclusions

Owing to the matchless set of conditioning factors, each human is unique and, despite all similarities, the transcriptomes of one person's cell phenotypes can never be identical with those of another person. In a profiled metastatic clear cell renal cell carcinoma [34], we found that even the transcriptomes of two cancer nodules isolated from the same kidney and categorized with the same Fuhrman grade 3 were largely different from each other. Moreover, some of the gene expression conditioning factors (environment, exposure to stress and toxins, medical treatment, diet, ageing etc.) are not constant, forcing the transcriptomes of cancer cells to continuously adapt. By consequence, the gene hierarchy is not only unique for each person and in each of his/her cancer nodules, but it changes over time. As such, this study provides strong reasons in favor of a really personalized and time-sensitive cancer gene therapy based on the manipulation of the gene master regulators.

Supplementary Materials: The following are available online at http://www.mdpi.com/2073-4425/11/9/1030/s1, Figure S1: GCH scores of the genes included in FoundationOne®CDx assay. The assay explores genes with full coding exonic regions for the detection of substitutions, insertion-deletions (indels), and copy-number alterations (CNAs), genes with select intronic regions for the detection of gene rearrangements, one gene with a promoter region and one non-coding RNA gene. Several genes (*BRAF, BRCA1, EGFR, FGFR1/3, KMT2A, MSH2, MYC. NOTCH2, RAF1, RARA*) have both exonic and intronic regions used for detection.

Funding: This research was supported by the Texas A&M University System Chancellor's Research Initiative (CRI) funding for the Center for Computational Systems Biology at the Prairie View A&M University.

Conflicts of Interest: The author declares no conflict of interest.

References

1. Cancer Org Portal. Available online: https://www.cancer.org/cancer/thyroid-cancer (accessed on 26 July 2020).
2. Thyroid Cancer Portal. Available online: https://www.thyroid.org/thyroid-cancer/ (accessed on 26 July 2020).
3. Cancer Gov. Available online: https://portal.gdc.cancer.gov (accessed on 26 July 2020).
4. 1000 Genomes Project Consortium; Auton, A.; Brooks, L.D.; Durbin, R.M.; Garrison, E.P.; Kang, H.M.; Korbel, J.O.; Marchini, J.L.; McCarthy, S.; McVean, G.A.; et al. A global reference for human genetic variation. *Nature* **2015**, *526*, 68–74. [CrossRef] [PubMed]
5. Alexander, E.K.; Kennedy, G.C.; Baloch, Z.W.; Cibas, E.S.; Chudova, D.; Diggans, J.; Friedman, L.; Kloos, R.T.; LiVolsi, V.A.; Mandel, S.J.; et al. Preoperative diagnosis of benign thyroid nodules with indeterminate cytology. *N. Engl. J. Med.* **2012**, *367*, 705–715. [CrossRef] [PubMed]
6. Abdullah, M.I.; Junit, S.M.; Ng, K.L.; Jayapalan, J.J.; Karikalan, B.; Hashim, O.H. Papillary Thyroid Cancer: Genetic Alterations and Molecular Biomrker Investigations. *Int. J. Med. Sci.* **2019**, *16*, 450–460. [CrossRef]
7. Foundation Medicine. Available online: https://www.foundationmedicine.com/genomic-testing (accessed on 12 July 2020).
8. Iacobas, D.A.; Tuli, N.; Iacobas, S.; Rasamny, J.K.; Moscatello, A.; Geliebter, J.; Tiwari, R.K. Gene master regulators of papillary and anaplastic thyroid cancer phenotypes. *Oncotarget* **2018**, *9*, 2410–2424. [CrossRef] [PubMed]
9. Iacobas, S.; Ede, N.; Iacobas, D.A. The Gene Master Regulators (GMR) Approach Provides Legitimate Targets for Personalized, Time-Sensitive Cancer Gene Therapy. *Genes* **2019**, *10*, 560. [CrossRef] [PubMed]
10. Iacobas, D.A. Commentary on "The Gene Master Regulators (GMR) Approach Provides Legitimate Targets for Personalized, Time-Sensitive Cancer Gene Therapy. *J. Cancer Immunol.* **2019**, *1*, 31–33. [CrossRef]
11. Iacobas, D.A. The Genomic Fabric Perspective on the Transcriptome between Universal Quantifiers and Personalized Genomic Medicine. *Biol. Theory* **2016**, *11*, 123–137. [CrossRef]
12. National Center for Biotechnology Information. Available online: https://www.ncbi.nlm.nih.gov/gds/?term=iacobas (accessed on 26 July 2020).

13. Zhang, H.; Xing, Z.; Mani, S.K.; Bancel, B.; Durantel, D.; Zoulim, F.; Tran, E.J.; Merle, P.; Andrisani, O. RNA helicase DEAD box protein 5 regulates Polycomb repressive complex 2/Hox transcript antisense intergenic RNA function in hepatitis B virus infection and hepatocarcinogenesis. *Hepatology* **2016**, *64*, 1033–1048. [CrossRef]
14. Liu, Y.; Tong, C.; Cao, J.; Xiong, M. NEMP1 Promotes Tamoxifen Resistance in Breast Cancer Cells. *Biochem. Genet.* **2019**, *57*, 813–826. [CrossRef]
15. Liu, Y.; Cheng, Z.; Li, Q.; Pang, Y.; Cui, L.; Qian, T.; Quan, L.; Dai, Y.; Jiao, Y.; Zhang, Z.; et al. Prognostic significance of the PANK family expression in acute myeloid leukemia. *Ann. Transl. Med.* **2019**, *7*, 261. [CrossRef]
16. Iacobas, D.A.; Iacobas, S.; Stout, R.; Spray, D.C. Cellular environment remodels the genomic fabrics of functional pathways in astrocytes. *Genes* **2020**, *11*, 520. [CrossRef]
17. Iacobas, D.A.; Iacobas, S.; Lee, P.R.; Cohen, J.E.; Fields, R.D. Coordinated Activity of Transcriptional Networks Responding to the Pattern of Action Potential Firing in Neurons. *Genes* **2019**, *10*, 754. [CrossRef] [PubMed]
18. Iacobas, D.A.; Iacobas, S.; Spray, D.C. Connexin43 and the brain transcriptome of the newborn mice. *Genomics* **2007**, *89*, 113–123. [CrossRef]
19. Mathew, R.; Huang, J.; Iacobas, S.; Iacobas, D.A. Pulmonary Hypertension Remodels the Genomic Fabrics of Major Functional Pathways. *Genes* **2020**, *11*, 126. [CrossRef] [PubMed]
20. Iacobas, D.A.; Iacobas, S.; Tanowitz, H.B.; de Carvalho, A.C.; Spray, D.C. Functional genomic fabrics are remodeled in a mouse model of Chagasic cardiomyopathy and restored following cell therapy. *Microbes Infect.* **2018**, *20*, 185–195. [CrossRef] [PubMed]
21. Kanehisa, M.; Furumichi, M.; Tanabe, M.; Sato, Y.; Morishima, K. KEGG: New perspectives on genomes, pathways, diseases and drugs. *Nucleic Acids Res.* **2017**, *45*, D353–D361. [CrossRef]
22. Kyoto Encyclopedia of Genes and Genomes. Available online: http://www.genome.jp/kegg/ (accessed on 21 June 2020).
23. Liu, Y.C.; Yeh, C.T.; Lin, K.H. Molecular Functions of Thyroid Hormone Signaling in Regulation of Cancer Progression and Anti-Apoptosis. *Int. J. Mol. Sci.* **2019**, *20*, 4986. [CrossRef]
24. Bai, J.W.; Wei, M.; Li, J.W.; Zhang, G.J. Notch Signaling Pathway and Endocrine Resistance in Breast Cancer. *Front. Pharmacol.* **2020**, *11*, 924. [CrossRef]
25. Yuan, Y.; Ju, Y.S.; Kim, Y.; Li, J.; Wang, Y.; Yoon, C.J.; Yang, Y.; Martincorena, I.; Creighton, C.J.; Weinstein, J.N.; et al. Comprehensive molecular characterization of mitochondrial genomes in human cancers. *Nat. Genet.* **2020**, *52*, 342–352. [CrossRef]
26. Kobawala, T.P.; Trivedi, T.I.; Gajjar, K.K.; Patel, D.H.; Patel, G.H.; Ghosh, N.R. Significance of Interleukin-6 in Papillary Thyroid Carcinoma. *J. Thyroid. Res.* **2016**, *2016*, 6178921. [CrossRef]
27. Bao, Y.; Zhao, T.L.; Zhang, Z.Q.; Liang, X.L.; Wang, Z.X.; Xiong, Y.; Lu, X.; Wang, L.H. High eukaryotic translation elongation factor 1 alpha 1 expression promotes proliferation and predicts poor prognosis in clear cell renal cell carcinoma. *Neoplasma* **2020**, *67*, 78–84. [CrossRef] [PubMed]
28. Wu, C.C.; Lin, J.D.; Chen, J.T.; Chang, C.M.; Weng, H.F.; Hsueh, C.; Chien, H.P.; Yu, J.S. Integrated analysis of fine-needle-aspiration cystic fluid proteome, cancer cell secretome, and public transcriptome datasets for papillary thyroid cancer biomarker discovery. *Oncotarget* **2018**, *9*, 12079–12100. [CrossRef] [PubMed]
29. Luo, D.; Chen, H.; Lu, P.; Li, X.; Long, M.; Peng, X.; Huang, M.; Huang, K.; Lin, S.; Tan, L.; et al. CHI3L1 overexpression is associated with metastasis and is an indicator of poor prognosis in papillary thyroid carcinoma. *Cancer Biomark.* **2017**, *18*, 273–284. [CrossRef] [PubMed]
30. Cheng, S.P.; Lee, J.J.; Chang, Y.C.; Lin, C.H.; Li, Y.S.; Liu, C.L. Overexpression of chitinase-3-like protein 1 is associated with structural recurrence in patients with differentiated thyroid cancer. *J. Pathol.* **2020**, e5503. [CrossRef]
31. Oczko-Wojciechowska, M.; Pfeifer, A.; Jarzab, M.; Swierniak, M.; Rusinek, D.; Tyszkiewicz, T.; Kowalska, M.; Chmielik, E.; Zembala-Nozynska, E.; Czarniecka, A.; et al. Impact of the Tumor Microenvironment on the Gene Expression Profile in Papillary Thyroid Cancer. *Pathobiology* **2020**, *87*, 143–154. [CrossRef] [PubMed]
32. Jevnikar, Z.; Rojnik, M.; Jamnik, P.; Doljak, B.; Fonovic, U.P.; Kos, J. Cathepsin H mediates the processing of talin and regulates migration of prostate cancer cells. *J. Biol. Chem.* **2013**, *288*, 2201–2209. [CrossRef]
33. Iacobas, D.A.; Iacobas, S.; Werner, P.; Scemes, E.; Spray, D.C. Alteration of transcriptomic networks in adoptive-transfer experimental autoimmune encephalomyelitis. *Front. Integr. Neurosci.* **2007**, *1*. [CrossRef]

34. Iacobas, D.A.; Iacobas, S. Towards a Personalized Cancer Gene Therapy: A Case of Clear Cell Renal Cell Carcinoma. *Cancer Oncol. Res.* **2017**, *5*, 45–52. [CrossRef]
35. Frigeri, A.; Iacobas, D.A.; Iacobas, S.; Nicchia, G.P.; Desaphy, J.-F.; Camerino, D.C.; Svelto, M.; Spray, D.C. Effect of microagravity on brain gene expression in mice. *Exp. Brain Res.* **2008**, *191*, 289–300. [CrossRef]
36. Iacobas, D.A.; Fan, C.; Iacobas, S.; Spray, D.C.; Haddad, G.G. Transcriptomic changes in developing kidney exposed to chronic hypoxia. *Biochem. Biophys. Res. Commun.* **2006**, *349*, 329–338. [CrossRef]
37. Iacobas, D.A.; Fan, C.; Iacobas, S.; Haddad, G.G. Integrated transcriptomic response to cardiac chronic hypoxia: Translation regulators and response to stress in cell survival. *Funct. Integr. Genom.* **2008**, *8*, 265–275. [CrossRef] [PubMed]
38. Iacobas, D.A.; Iacobas, S.; Haddad, G.G. Heart rhythm genomic fabric in hypoxia. *Biochem. Biophys. Res. Commun.* **2010**, *391*, 1769–1774. [CrossRef] [PubMed]
39. Iacobas, D.A.; Urban, M.; Iacobas, S.; Scemes, E.; Spray, D.C. Array analysis of gene expression in connexin43 null astrocytes. *Physiol. Genom.* **2003**, *15*, 177–190. [CrossRef] [PubMed]
40. Iacobas, D.A.; Iacobas, S.; Urban-Maldonado, M.; Scemes, E.; Spray, D.C. Similar transcriptomic alterations in Cx43 knock-down and knock-out astrocytes. *Cell Commun. Adhes.* **2008**, *15*, 195–206. [CrossRef] [PubMed]
41. Surmiak, M.; Hubalewska-Mazgaj, M.; Wawrzycka-Adamczyk, K.; Musiał, J.; Sanak, M. Delayed neutrophil apoptosis in granulomatosis with polyangiitis: Dysregulation of neutrophil gene signature and circulating apoptosis-related proteins. *Scand. J. Rheumatol.* **2020**, *49*, 57–67. [CrossRef]
42. Zhao, Y.; Liu, X.; Zhong, L.; He, M.; Chen, S.; Wang, T.; Ma, S. The combined use of miRNAs and mRNAs as biomarkers for the diagnosis of papillary thyroid carcinoma. *Int. J. Mol. Med.* **2015**, *36*, 1097–1103. [CrossRef]
43. Deligiorgi, M.V.; Mahaira, H.; Eftychiadis, C.; Kafiri, G.; Georgiou, G.; Theodoropoulos, G.; Konstadoulakis, M.M.; Zografos, E.; Zografos, G.C. RANKL, OPG, TRAIL, KRas, and c-Fos expression in relation to central lymph node metastases in papillary thyroid carcinoma. *J. BU ON Off. J. Balk. Union Oncol.* **2018**, *23*, 1029–1040.
44. Kataki, A.; Sotirianakos, S.; Memos, N.; Karayiannis, M.; Messaris, E.; Leandros, E.; Manouras, A.; Androulakis, G. P53 and C-FOS overexpression in patients with thyroid cancer: An immunohistochemical study. *Neoplasma* **2003**, *50*, 26–30.
45. Franceschi, S.; Lessi, F.; Panebianco, F.; Tantillo, E.; La Ferla, M.; Menicagli, M.; Aretini, P.; Apollo, A.; Naccarato, A.G.; Marchetti, I.; et al. Loss of c-KIT expression in thyroid cancer cells. *PLoS ONE* **2017**, *12*, e0173913. [CrossRef]
46. Chu, Y.H.; Sadow, P.M. Noninvasive Follicular Thyroid Neoplasm with Papillary-Like Nuclear Features (NIFTP): Diagnostic Updates and Molecular Advances. In *Seminars in Diagnostic Pathology*; WB Saunders: Philadelphia, PA, USA, 2020.
47. Lubos, E.; Kelly, N.J.; Oldebeken, S.R.; Leopold, J.A.; Zhang, Y.Y.; Loscalzo, J.; Handy, D.E. Glutathione peroxidase-1 deficiency augments proinflammatory cytokine-induced redox signaling and human endothelial cell activation. *J. Biol. Chem.* **2011**, *286*, 35407–35417. [CrossRef]
48. Cardoso, M.F.S.; Castelletti, C.H.M.; Lima-Filho, J.L.; Martins, D.B.G.; Teixeira, J.A.C. Putative biomarkers for cervical cancer: SNVs, methylation and expression profiles. *Mutat. Res.* **2017**, *773*, 161–173. [CrossRef] [PubMed]
49. Mei, L.; Shen, C.; Miao, R.; Wang, J.Z.; Cao, M.D.; Zhang, Y.S.; Shi, L.H.; Zhao, G.H.; Wang, M.H.; Wu, L.S.; et al. RNA methyltransferase NSUN2 promotes gastric cancer cell proliferation by repressing p57Kip2 by an m5C-dependent manner. *Cell Death Dis.* **2020**, *11*, 270. [CrossRef] [PubMed]
50. Matsuda, S.; Murakami, M.; Ikeda, Y.; Nakagawa, Y.; Tsuji, A.; Kitagishi, Y. Role of tumor suppressor molecules in genomic perturbations and damaged DNA repair involved in the pathogenesis of cancer and neurodegeneration (Review). *Biomed. Rep.* **2020**, *13*, 10. [CrossRef]
51. Księżakowska-Łakoma, K.; Żyła, M.; Wilczyński, J.R. Mitochondrial dysfunction in cancer. *Prz. Menopauzalny* **2014**, *13*, 136–144. [CrossRef]
52. Huang, Y.P.; Chang, N.W. PPARα modulates gene expression profiles of mitochondrial energy metabolism in oral tumorigenesis. *Biomedicine* **2016**, *6*, 3. [CrossRef]
53. Roversi, F.M.; Olalla Saad, S.T.; Machado-Neto, J.A. Serine peptidase inhibitor Kunitz type 2 (SPINT2) in cancer development and progression. *Biomed. Pharmacother.* **2018**, *101*, 278–286. [CrossRef]
54. Guan, X.; Guan, Z.; Song, C. Expression profile analysis identifies key genes as prognostic markers for metastasis of osteosarcoma. *Cancer Cell Int.* **2020**, *20*, 104. [CrossRef]

55. Graumann, J.; Finkernagel, F.; Reinartz, S.; Stief, T.; Brödje, D.; Renz, H.; Jansen, J.M.; Wagner, U.; Worzfeld, T.; Pogge von Strandmann, E.; et al. Multi-platform affinity proteomics identify proteins linked to metastasis and immune suppression in ovarian cancer plasma. *Front. Oncol.* **2019**, *9*, 1150. [CrossRef] [PubMed]
56. Liu, F.; Cox, C.D.; Chowdhury, R.; Dovek, L.; Nguyen, H.; Li, T.; Li, S.; Ozer, B.; Chou, A.; Nguyen, N.; et al. SPINT2 is hypermethylated in both IDH1 mutated and wild-type glioblastomas, and exerts tumor suppression via reduction of c-Met activation. *J. Neurooncol.* **2019**, *142*, 423–434. [CrossRef] [PubMed]
57. Pereira, M.S.; Celeiro, S.P.; Costa, Â.M.; Pinto, F.; Popov, S.; de Almeida, G.C.; Amorim, J.; Pires, M.M.; Pinheiro, C.; Lopes, J.M.; et al. Loss of SPINT2 expression frequently occurs in glioma, leading to increased growth and invasion via MMP2. *Cell. Oncol.* **2020**, *43*, 107–121. [CrossRef] [PubMed]
58. Wu, L.; Shu, X.; Bao, J.; Guo, X.; Kote-Jarai, Z.; Haiman, C.A.; Eeles, R.A.; Zheng, W.; PRACTICAL, CRUK, BPC3, CAPS, PEGASUS Consortia. Analysis of Over 140,000 European Descendants Identifies Genetically Predicted Blood Protein Biomarkers Associated with Prostate Cancer Risk. *Cancer Res.* **2019**, *79*, 4592–4598. [CrossRef] [PubMed]
59. Ma, Z.; Liu, D.; Li, W.; Di, S.; Zhang, Z.; Zhang, J.; Xu, L.; Guo, K.; Zhu, Y.; Han, J.; et al. STYK1 promotes tumor growth and metastasis by reducing SPINT2/HAI-2 expression in non-small cell lung cancer. *Cell Death Dis.* **2019**, *10*, 435. [CrossRef] [PubMed]
60. Roversi, F.M.; Cury, N.M.; Lopes, M.R.; Ferro, K.P.; Machado-Neto, J.A.; Alvarez, M.C.; Dos Santos, G.P.; Giardini Rosa, R.; Longhini, A.L.; Duarte, A.D.S.S.; et al. Up-regulation of SPINT2/HAI-2 by Azacytidine in bone marrow mesenchymal stromal cells affects leukemic stem cell survival and adhesion. *J. Cell. Mol. Med.* **2019**, *23*, 1562–1571. [CrossRef] [PubMed]
61. Wang, N.; Che, Y.; Yin, F.; Yu, F.; Bi, X.; Wang, Y. Study on the methylation status of SPINT2 gene and its expression in cervical carcinoma. *Cancer Biomark.* **2018**, *22*, 435–442. [CrossRef] [PubMed]
62. Rodríguez, C.F.; Llorca, O. RPAP3 C-Terminal Domain: A Conserved Domain for the Assembly of R2TP Co-Chaperone Complexes. *Cells* **2020**, *9*, 1139. [CrossRef] [PubMed]
63. Kawachi, T.; Tanaka, S.; Fukuda, A.; Sumii, Y.; Setiawan, A.; Kotoku, N.; Kobayashi, M.; Arai, M. Target identification of the marine natural products Dictyoceratin-A and -C as selective growth inhibitors in cancer cells adapted to hypoxic environments. *Mar. Drugs* **2019**, *17*, 163. [CrossRef]
64. Liu, F.; Zhao, H.; Gong, L.; Yao, L.; Li, Y.; Zhang, W. MicroRNA-129-3p functions as a tumor suppressor in serous ovarian cancer by targeting BZW1. *Int. J. Clin. Exp. Pathol.* **2018**, *11*, 5901–5908.
65. Chiou, J.; Chang, Y.C.; Jan, Y.H.; Tsai, H.F.; Yang, C.J.; Huang, M.S.; Yu, Y.L.; Hsiao, M. Overexpression of BZW1 is an independent poor prognosis marker and its down-regulation suppresses lung adenocarcinoma metastasis. *Sci. Rep.* **2019**, *9*, 14624. [CrossRef]
66. Li, S.; Chai, Z.; Li, Y.; Liu, D.; Bai, Z.; Li, Y.; Li, Y.; Situ, Z. BZW1, a novel proliferation regulator that promotes growth of salivary muocepodermoid carcinoma. *Cancer Lett.* **2009**, *284*, 86–94. [CrossRef]
67. Iacobas, D.A.; Iacobas, S.; Spray, D.C. Connexin-dependent transcellular transcriptomic networks in mouse brain. *Prog. Biophys. Mol. Biol.* **2007**, *94*, 168–184. [CrossRef]

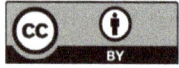

© 2020 by the author. Licensee MDPI, Basel, Switzerland. This article is an open access article distributed under the terms and conditions of the Creative Commons Attribution (CC BY) license (http://creativecommons.org/licenses/by/4.0/).

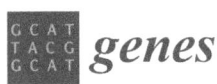

Article

Association between Family Histories of Thyroid Cancer and Thyroid Cancer Incidence: A Cross-Sectional Study Using the Korean Genome and Epidemiology Study Data

Soo-Hwan Byun [1,2], Chanyang Min [3], Hyo-Geun Choi [2,3,4,*] and Seok-Jin Hong [2,5,*]

1. Department of Oral & Maxillofacial Surgery, Dentistry, Hallym University College of Medicine, Anyang 14068, Korea; purheit@daum.net
2. Research Center of Clinical Dentistry, Hallym University Clinical Dentistry Graduate School, Chuncheon 24252, Korea
3. Hallym Data Science Laboratory, Hallym University College of Medicine, Anyang 14068, Korea; joicemin@naver.com
4. Department of Otorhinolaryngology-Head & Neck Surgery, Hallym University College of Medicine, Anyang 14068, Korea
5. Department of Otorhinolaryngology-Head & Neck Surgery, Hallym University College of Medicine, Dongtan 18450, Korea
* Correspondence: pupen@naver.com (H.-G.C.); enthsj@hanmail.net (S.-J.H.); Tel.: +82-10-9033-9224 (H.-G.C.); +82-31-8086-2670 (S.-J.H.)

Received: 28 July 2020; Accepted: 1 September 2020; Published: 3 September 2020

Abstract: This study assessed the association between thyroid cancer and family history. This cross-sectional study used epidemiological data from the Korean Genome and Epidemiology Study from 2001 to 2013. Among 211,708 participants, 988 were in the thyroid cancer group and 199,588 were in the control group. Trained interviewers questioned the participants to obtain their thyroid cancer history and age at onset. The participants were examined according to their age, sex, monthly household income, obesity, smoking, alcohol consumption, and past medical history. The adjusted odds ratios (95% confidence intervals) for the family histories of fathers, mothers, and siblings were 6.59 (2.05–21.21), 4.76 (2.59–8.74), and 9.53 (6.92–13.11), respectively, and were significant. The results for the subgroup analyses according to sex were consistent. The rate of family histories of thyroid cancer for fathers and siblings were not different according to the thyroid cancer onset, while that of mothers were higher in participants with a younger age at onset (<50 years old group, 11/523 [2.1%], $p = 0.007$). This study demonstrated that thyroid cancer incidence was associated with thyroid cancer family history. This supports regular examination of individuals with a family history of thyroid cancer to prevent disease progression and ensure early management.

Keywords: epidemiology; thyroid cancer; family history; differentiated thyroid cancer; papillary thyroid cancer

1. Introduction

The incidence of thyroid cancer is increasing worldwide [1], and it has increased by approximately two folds over the past few decades [2]. The incidence of thyroid nodules diagnosed by palpation of the thyroid gland is approximately 5–10% in adults [3]. Because of the frequent use and accessibility of thyroid ultrasonography (US), there has been an increase in thyroid cancer detection [4]. The objective of the examination of patients with thyroid nodules is to identify thyroid cancer. As a result, its incidence in South Korea in 2011 was 15 times higher than in 1993 [5]. Korean women had the highest age-standardized incidence of thyroid cancer globally [6]. Differentiated thyroid carcinoma (DTC) comprises approximately 90% of all thyroid cancers and includes the papillary type and follicular type [7,8]. In Korea, the most common histological type (94.9%) of DTC is papillary thyroid cancer (PTC) [9]. Total thyroidectomy is usually recommended for treatment of thyroid cancer, followed by radioiodine therapy in some cases. Inoperable or radiotherapy refractory differentiated thyroid cancers are commonly the main causes of thyroid cancer-related deaths and do not have effective treatments [10]. Cytotoxic chemotherapy with innovative medicines should be studied because they appear to be effective in some patients [11,12].

The etiology of DTC is still unknown. However, environmental and genetic predisposing factors including ionizing radiation might affect the development of thyroid cancer [13]. Air pollution and iodine intake are considered risk factors for thyroid cancer [14–17]. Obesity, smoking, and alcohol consumption are also associated with thyroid cancer [18]. A family history of thyroid cancer is also a suggested risk factor in 5–15% of cases. There are several genetic mutations identified to have a role in the development of DTC [7]. Rearranged during transfection (RET) chromosomal rearrangement genes, and mutation of RAS or BRAF proto-oncogenes can trigger the activation of the mitogen-activated protein kinase cascade in PTC. Mutations of the BRAF, RAS, or RET genes are found in nearly 70% of PTC cases [19,20]. A previous study mentioned that BRAF mutation is associated with aggressiveness of PTC and the loss of radiotherapy effectiveness in recurrent disease. Surgical resection of mutation-positive cancer is recommended [10]. For instance, lobectomy is recommended by the American Thyroid Association for treatment of PTCs < 1 cm [21]. However, because of the definite association of BRAF mutation with aggressiveness of PTC, total thyroidectomy might be a better treatment option if BRAF mutation is positive in preoperative testing [21].

The familial risk of thyroid cancer is known to be highest in all cancer sites, for which the increased risk extends beyond the nuclear family [22–24]. Family history is a possible risk factor which could be associated with medical and psychosocial benefits. To provide definite information, the clinicians and entire medical system need to recognize the familial risks that are not included in the conventional familial risk guidelines.

Nevertheless, only few studies have studied the risk factors of familial history for thyroid cancer in Asian adults. Most of the studies were focused on familial non-medullary thyroid cancer, or the study sample sizes were relatively small [25]. Myung et al. reported that a family history of cancer and alcohol consumption were associated with a decreased risk of thyroid cancer, whereas a higher body mass index (BMI) and family history of thyroid cancer were associated with an increased risk of thyroid cancer in 34,211 patients [26]. The study was a case-control study. A total of 802 thyroid cancer cases out of 34,211 patients was included. A total of 802 control cases was also selected from the same cohort group and matched using the ratio 1:1 by age and area of residence. Multivariate conditional logistic regression analysis was used. The results show that females and those with a family history of thyroid cancer had an increased risk of thyroid cancer, and a family history of cancer and alcohol consumption were associated with a decreased risk of thyroid cancer, whereas a higher BMI and family history of thyroid cancer were associated with an increased risk of thyroid cancer. The study suggested that females and those with a family history of thyroid cancer have an increased risk of thyroid cancer. Hwang et al. showed that multicollinearity existed between US assessment and patient age, and first-degree family history of thyroid cancer and serum thyroid hormone values in 1254 patients [25]. A retrospective study investigated 1310 thyroid nodules of 1254 euthyroid asymptomatic patients who underwent US-guided fine needle aspiration. The study evaluated nodule size, first-degree family history of thyroid cancer, gender, age, and thyroid-stimulating hormone (TSH) levels with US examination to distinguish between benign and malignant nodules. Multiple logistic regression analysis was conducted to evaluate the risk of thyroid malignancy according to clinical and US features. A first-degree family history of thyroid cancer, age, and high TSH levels did not independently significantly increase the risk of thyroid cancer. The study concluded that a first-degree family history as a risk factor for thyroid malignancy should be further investigated in asymptomatic patients.

Similar to those studies, previous studies of familial risk were performed without a control group or with a small control group. Moreover, those studies did not include many confounding factors that could influence the study results. To the best of our knowledge, there has been no study on the association between family history and thyroid cancer using large Korean population data.

A clear picture of the association between thyroid cancer and family history will help both patients and clinicians. This could serve as a basis for guidelines governing clinical risk factor assessment and the management of thyroid nodules. Therefore, this study assessed the association between thyroid cancer and family history.

2. Materials and Methods

2.1. Study Population and Data Collection

Authorization was obtained from the ethics committee of the Hallym University (2019-02-020). The requirement for written informed consent was waived by the Institutional Review Board. This cross-sectional study relied on the data from the Korean Genome and Epidemiology Study (KoGES) from 2001 to 2013.

The Korean Genome and Epidemiology Study Health Examinee (KoGES HEXA) is a large cohort project initiated to reveal gene-environmental factors and their interactions in diseases [27,28]. Among this, we have selected the questionnaires. Therefore, this study had a cross-sectional design. KoGES was designed to identify gene-environment factors and their interactions in common chronic diseases, such as hypertension, cardiovascular disease, type 2 diabetes, obesity, and metabolic syndrome, in Korea. KoGES collected epidemiological data and biospecimens, such as urine, blood, and genome, from many patients aged 40–69 years by performing a medical examination and health survey. Familial data were well-organized and systemized, and the data were collected using a questionnaire, which was confirmed by expert clinicians. The KoGES data were collected from both urban and rural areas. Therefore, the study sample size was relatively larger than that reported in previous studies.

2.2. Participant Selection

Among 211,708 participants, we excluded the participants with no family history of thyroid cancer ($n = 10,030$) and no BMI data ($n = 1102$) (Figure 1). In total, 200,576 participants (69,693 men, 130,883 women) were evaluated. According to their cancer thyroid histories, they were divided into two groups: the thyroid cancer group and control group.

2.3. Survey

Trained interviewers asked the participants questions to obtain relevant data including previous thyroid cancer history, age at onset, household monthly income, past metabolic disease history (hypertension, diabetes mellitus, and hyperlipidemia), smoking history, and alcohol consumption history. Anthropometric and clinical measurements were obtained [27,28]. This study categorized the family histories of thyroid cancer into groups: fathers, mothers, and siblings (brothers or sisters). Income was categorized into four groups according to the household monthly income: no information, low (<$1500), middle (≥$1500–<$3000), and high (≥$3000). BMI was used to measure obesity (kg/m^2), wherein height and weight were considered as continuous variables [27,29]. Total smoking histories were calculated in pack-year, and alcohol consumption was measured as the mean daily alcohol consumption (g/day) using the frequency and alcohol types [30,31].

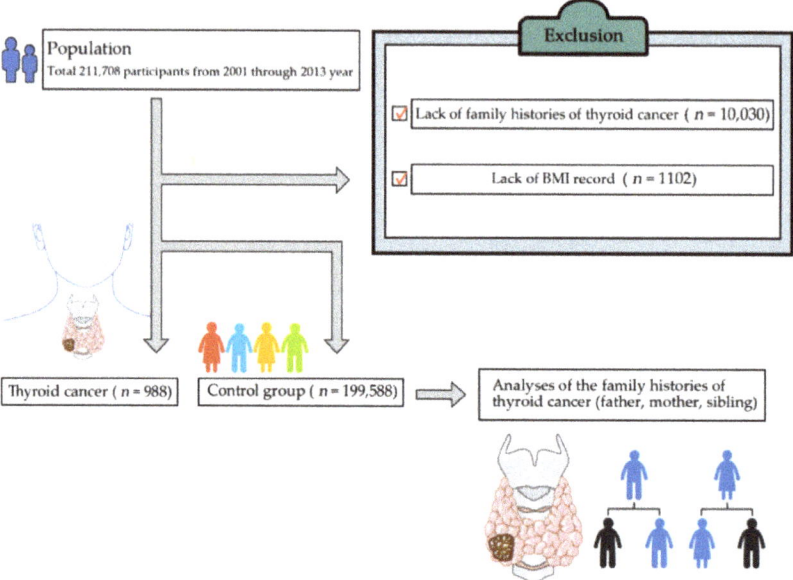

Figure 1. Participant selection.

2.4. Statistical Analyses

The chi-square test or Fisher's exact test was used to compare the differences between sex, income, metabolic disease history, and thyroid cancer family history between both groups. The independent *t*-test was used to compare the age, BMI, smoking pack year, and alcohol consumption.

To analyze the odds ratio (OR) of thyroid cancer history for the thyroid cancer group, a logistic regression model was used. In the crude model, this study only inserted each family history of thyroid cancer as an independent variable. In Model 1, this study inserted each family history of thyroid cancer and age, sex, income, BMI, smoking, alcohol intake, and past medical histories of hypertension, diabetes mellitus, and dyslipidemia as independent variables. In Model 2, this study inserted thyroid cancer history of the father, mother, and siblings as independent variables. In Model 3, this study inserted the variables of Models 2 and 3. To analyze the interaction between the different family histories of thyroid cancer, we designed Model 4. In this model, the variables included: thyroid cancer history of father, mother, siblings, father × siblings, and mother × siblings.

The 95% confidence intervals (CIs) were calculated. For the subgroup analysis, this study stratified the participants according to sex: male and female.

Two-tailed analyses were conducted, and *p* values < 0.05 were considered as statistically significant. The results were analyzed using SPSS v. 22.0 (IBM, Armonk, NY, USA).

3. Results

The participant age ranged from 40 to 91 years. In total, 988 participants were in the thyroid cancer group, while 199,588 were in the control group. The differences between the mean age, BMI, smoking duration, and daily alcohol consumption of both groups were significant (Table 1). The rates of sex, income, past medical history of diabetes mellitus, and dyslipidemia were also different between both groups.

Table 1. General characteristics of participants.

Characteristics	Total Participants		p-Value
	Thyroid Cancer (n, %)	Control (n, %)	
Total number (n, %)	988 (100.0)	199,588 (100.0)	
Age (years, mean, SD)	53.2 (7.6)	53.9 (8.7)	0.007 [1]
Sex (n, %)			<0.001 [1]
Male	79 (8.0)	69,614 (34.9)	
Female	909 (92.0)	129,974 (65.1)	
Income (n, %)			<0.001 [1]
No information	95 (9.6)	40,590 (20.3)	
Low	166 (16.8)	41,060 (20.6)	
Middle	292 (29.6)	51,899 (26.0)	
High	435 (44.0)	66,039 (33.1)	
Hypertension (n, %)	220 (22.3)	40,930 (20.5)	0.172
Diabetes (n, %)	50 (5.1)	14,584 (7.3)	0.007 [1]
Dyslipidemia (n, %)	117 (11.8)	17,834 (8.9)	0.001 [1]
Obesity (BMI, kg/m^2, mean, SD)	23.8 (2.9)	24.0 (3.0)	<0.001 [1]
Tobacco index (pack-year, mean, SD)	1.63 (6.5)	6.62 (12.5)	<0.001 [1]
alcohol consumption (g/day, mean, SD)	2.0 (10.1)	7.2 (22.1)	<0.001 [1]
Family history of father (n, %)	3 (0.3)	86 (0.0)	0.010 [1]
Family history of mother (n, %)	12 (1.2)	307 (0.2)	<0.001 [1]
Family history of siblings (n, %)	44 (4.5)	653 (0.3)	<0.001 [1]

BMI, body mass index, kg/m^2; SD, Standard deviation. [1] Independent t-test, Chi-square test, or Fisher's exact test. Significance at $p < 0.05$.

In Model 1, adjusted for general characteristics, the adjusted ORs for the family histories of fathers, mothers, and siblings were 6.72 (95% CI = 2.10–21.50), 6.33 (95% CI = 3.52–11.36), and 10.16 (95% CI = 7.42–13.93), respectively.

In Model 2, adjusted for only family histories of thyroid cancer, the adjusted ORs for family histories of fathers, mothers, and siblings were 6.75 (95% CI = 2.10–21.67), 5.55 (95% CI = 3.02–10.19), and 13.09 (95% CI = 9.53–17.99), respectively.

In Model 3, adjusted for both general characteristics and family histories of thyroid cancer, the adjusted OR was slightly lower than in Models 1 and 2. The adjusted ORs for the family histories of fathers, mothers, and siblings were 6.59 (95% CI = 2.05–21.21), 4.76 (95% CI = 2.59–8.74), and 9.53 (95% CI = 6.92–13.11), respectively, and were significant (Table 2).

Table 2. Association between thyroid cancer history and their family thyroid cancer histories.

Family History	ORs of Thyroid Cancer for the Thyroid Cancer Family Histories							
	Crude	p-Value	Model 1	p-Value	Model 2	p-Value	Model 3	p-Value
ORs of the thyroid cancer history of father								
Thyroid cancer	7.07 (2.23–22.38)	0.001 [1]	6.72 (2.10–21.50)	0.001 [1]	6.75 (2.10–21.67)	0.001 [1]	6.59 (2.05–21.21)	0.002 [1]
Control	1.00		1.00		1.00		1.00	
ORs of the thyroid cancer history of mother								
Thyroid cancer	7.98 (4.47–14.26)	<0.001 [1]	6.33 (3.52–11.36)	<0.001 [1]	5.55 (3.02–10.19)	<0.001 [1]	4.76 (2.59–8.74)	<0.001 [1]
Control	1.00		1.00		1.00		1.00	
ORs of the thyroid cancer history of siblings								
Thyroid cancer	14.20 (10.40–19.40)	<0.001 [1]	10.16 (7.42–13.93)	<0.001 [1]	13.09 (9.53–17.99)	<0.001 [1]	9.53 (6.92–13.11)	<0.001 [1]
Control	1.00		1.00		1.00		1.00	

ORs, odds ratios. Model 1: adjusted for age, sex, income, body mass index, smoking, alcohol intake, and past medical histories of hypertension, diabetes mellitus, and dyslipidemia. Model 2: adjusted for thyroid cancer history of father, mother, and siblings. Model 3: adjusted for Models 1 and 2. [1] Logistic regression analyses, Statistical significance at $p < 0.05$.

In the subgroup analyses according to sex, the results were consistent with the results of the total participants (Table 3). In men, the adjusted ORs for the family histories of fathers and siblings were 29.09 (95% CI = 3.84–220.29) and 14.15 (95% CI = 3.39–58.95), respectively, in Model 3, while that of mother did not converge. In women, the adjusted ORs for the family histories of fathers, mothers, and siblings were 4.71 (95% CI = 1.13–19.52), 5.06 (95% CI = 2.75–9.31) and 9.37 (95% CI = 6.75–13.00), respectively.

Table 3. Subgroup analyses of association between thyroid cancer history and their family thyroid cancer histories according to sex.

Family History	ORs of Thyroid Cancer for the Thyroid Cancer Histories of Families							
	Crude	p-Value	Model 1	p-Value	Model 2	p-Value	Model 3	p-Value
Men (n = 69,693)								
ORs of the thyroid cancer history of father								
Thyroid cancer	27.88 (3.76–206.55)	0.001 [1]	28.21 (3.73–213.69)	0.001 [1]	28.53 (3.85–211.44)	0.001 [1]	29.09 (3.84–220.29)	0.001 [1]
Control	1.00		1.00		1.00		1.00	
ORs of the thyroid cancer history of mother								
Thyroid cancer	No convergence	0.997	No convergence	0.997	No convergence	0.997	No convergence	0.997
Control	1.00		1.00		1.00		1.00	
ORs of the thyroid cancer history of siblings								
Thyroid cancer	15.43 (3.75–63.54)	<0.001 [1]	13.90 (3.34–57.94)	<0.001 [1]	16.02 (3.89–66.00)	<0.001 [1]	14.15 (3.39–58.95)	<0.001 [1]
Control	1.00		1.00		1.00		1.00	
Women (n = 130,883)								
ORs of the thyroid cancer history of father								
Thyroid cancer	5.31 (1.29–21.79)	0.021 [1]	4.84 (1.18–19.94)	0.029 [1]	4.92 (1.18–20.61)	0.029 [1]	4.71 (1.13–19.52)	0.033 [1]
Control	1.00		1.00		1.00		1.00	
ORs of the thyroid cancer history of mother								
Thyroid cancer	7.89 (4.40–14.16)	<0.001 [1]	6.75 (3.75–12.14)	<0.001 [1]	5.70 (3.09–10.51)	<0.001 [1]	5.06 (2.75–9.31)	<0.001 [1]
Control	1.00		1.00		1.00		1.00	
ORs of the thyroid cancer history of siblings								
Thyroid cancer	11.70 (8.49–16.13)	<0.001 [1]	10.04 (7.27–13.87)	<0.001 [1]	10.81 (7.80–14.98)	<0.001 [1]	9.37 (6.75–13.00)	<0.001 [1]
Control	1.00		1.00		1.00		1.00	

Model 1: adjusted for age, sex, income, body mass index, smoking, alcohol intake, and past medical histories of hypertension, diabetes mellitus, and dyslipidemia. Model 2: adjusted for thyroid cancer history of father, thyroid cancer history of mother, and thyroid cancer history of siblings. Model 3: adjusted for Models 1 and 2. [1] Logistic regression analyses, Statistical significance at $p < 0.05$.

Because no father had a thyroid cancer history when mother had thyroid cancer, we did not make the interaction model for father × mother. In the interaction model, we did not find any interaction in father × siblings and mother × siblings (Table 4).

Table 4. Interaction model of each family history of thyroid cancer.

Variable	ORs for Thyroid Cancer	
	Model 4	p-Value
Father	No convergence	1.00
Mother	12.84 (2.02–81.86)	0.007
Siblings	26.87 (5.69–126.91)	<0.001
Father × siblings	No convergence	1.000
Mother × siblings	0.51 (0.12–2.17)	0.362

Model 4: adjusted for thyroid cancer history of father, mother, siblings, father × siblings, and mother × siblings.

The rate of family histories of thyroid cancer of father and siblings were not different according to thyroid cancer onset (Table 5), while that of mother was higher in patients with a younger age at onset (<50 years group, 11/523 [2.1%]) compared with those with an older age at onset (≥50 years group, 1/456 [0.2%], $p = 0.007$).

Table 5. Ratio of family histories of thyroid cancer according to thyroid cancer onset among the thyroid cancer participants.

Histories	Onset of Thyroid Cancer		p-Value
	<50 Years Old	≥50 Years Old	
Thyroid cancer histories of father (n, %)			
Yes	3 (0.6)	0 (0.0)	0.253
No	520 (99.4)	456 (100.0)	
Thyroid cancer histories of mother (n, %)			
Yes	11 (2.1)	1 (0.2)	0.007 [1]
No	512 (97.9)	455 (99.8)	
Thyroid cancer histories of siblings (n, %)			
Yes	23 (4.4)	21 (4.6)	0.876
No	500 (95.6)	435 (95.4)	

[1] Fisher's exact test. Significance at $p < 0.05$.

4. Discussion

The definite association between family history and thyroid cancer incidence is not yet completely known. Although most cases of PTC occur sporadically, it seems that there are family components in some cases of PTC. Familial non-medullary thyroid cancer (FNMTC) is defined as a condition in which two or more first-degree relatives are affected by thyroid cancer in the absence of a known familial syndrome [32,33]. FNMTC shows a tendency to be more aggressive than sporadic cases with higher rates of extra-thyroid extension, lymph node metastases, larger tumor size in younger patients, and worse prognosis [32,33]. This study focused on the family history of PTC in a large population and not FNMTC. The most common histological type (94.9%) of DTC in Korea was PTC [9]. Most participants with thyroid cancer in the KoGES data would have PTC based on the results of previous studies [9,34–36]. There are few studies on the family history of PTC in a large population. Therefore, this study investigated the association between thyroid cancer and family history using data from a large Korean study.

This study showed that the adjusted OR for family history was higher in all thyroid cancer patients than in the control group (Table 2). Family history was significantly associated with the incidence of thyroid cancer after adjustment for age, sex, income, hypertension, diabetes, dyslipidemia, obesity, smoking, and alcohol consumption (Table 1). A meta-analysis of seven cohort studies by Zhao et al. showed that obesity increased the risk of thyroid cancer [37]. The meta-analysis evaluated the association between body weight or BMI and risk of thyroid cancer. A total of 5154 thyroid cancer cases was included. The pooled relative risk (RR) of thyroid cancer was 1.13 (95% CI 1.04–1.22) for overweight. Obesity was related with increased thyroid cancer risk in both genders, the strength of the association increasing with increasing BMI. The combined RR of thyroid cancer was 1.18 (95% CI 1.11–1.25) for excess body weight. Being overweight was associated with a significant increase in the thyroid cancer risk among non-Asians, but not among Asians. Overweight, obesity, and excess body weight were linked to PTC risk. Han et al. reported that obesity was associated with a higher prevalence of thyroid cancer in women [38]. The study collected data from 15,068 subjects who received a health examination from 2007 to 2008 at the Health Screening and Promotion Center of Asan Medical Center in Korea. Thyroid US was conducted in the examination, and suspected nodules were additionally examined by US-guided aspiration. Those with a history of thyroid disease or family history of thyroid cancer were excluded from the study. In total, 15,068 participants were screened by thyroid US. The prevalence of thyroid cancer in females was related with a high BMI (per 5 kg/m^2 increase) (OR = 1.63, 95% CI 1.24–2.10, $p < 0.001$) after adjustment for age, smoking status, and TSH levels. There was no significant correlation between the prevalence of thyroid cancer in males and a high BMI (OR = 1.16, 95% CI 0.85–1.57, $p = 0.336$). There was no association between age, fasting serum insulin, or basal TSH levels and thyroid cancer in either gender. In a meta-analysis of observational studies, Cho et al. showed that the risk of thyroid cancer was decreased by 21% in smokers compared to non-smokers [39]. The study investigated 31 studies to analyze the relationship between thyroid cancer occurrence and smoking. These studies consisted of 6260 thyroid cancer cases and 32,935 controls. The cohort studies included 2715 thyroid cancer patients. Summary RRs and 95% CIs were calculated using a random effects model. The risk of thyroid cancer was decreased in participants with a past smoking history (RR = 0.79; 95% CI 0.70–0.88) compared with those without. However, strong evidence of heterogeneity was found among the investigated studies; therefore, subgroup analyses were performed according to study location, study type, source of controls, smoking status, sex, and histological type of thyroid cancer. When the data were stratified by smoking status, an inverse association was observed only among current smokers (RR = 0.74; 95% CI 0.64–0.86), not former smokers (RR = 1.01; 95% CI 0.92–1.10). Previous studies demonstrated that alcohol consumption was found to be significantly associated with a decreased risk of thyroid cancer when the analysis was performed using the control group [40–42]. Kitahara et al. evaluated data from five prospective United States studies (384,433 males and 361,664 females) [40]. Hazard ratios and 95% CIs for thyroid cancer were calculated from adjusted models of smoking and alcohol consumption with additional adjustment of age, sex, race, education, and BMI. In total, 1003 thyroid cancer cases (335 males and 668 females) were identified. Alcohol intake was also inversely associated with thyroid cancer risk (≥7 drinks/week versus 0, HR = 0.72, 95% CI 0.58–0.90). Inverse associations with alcohol consumption were more pronounced for papillary versus follicular tumors. Hong et al. investigated 33 observational studies with two cross-sectional studies, 20 case-control studies, and 11 cohort studies [42]. The studies involved 7725 thyroid cancer participants and 3,113,679 participants without thyroid cancer. In the fixed-effect model meta-analysis of all 33 studies, alcohol intake was related with a reduced risk of thyroid cancer (OR = 0.74; 95% CI 0.67–0.83). In the subgroup meta-analysis, alcohol consumption also reduced the risk of thyroid cancer in both case-control studies (OR = 0.77; 95% CI 0.65–0.92) and cohort studies (RR = 0.70; 95% CI 0.60–0.82). Subgroup meta-analyses showed that alcohol consumption was significantly related with a reduced risk of thyroid cancer.

The present study adjusted for various confounding factors to reduce the surveillance bias. The adjusted ORs in this study were similar to those in previous studies performed in other countries [7,8,23]. Kust et al. reported that family history plays a significant role in the development of thyroid cancer. Having first-degree relatives with thyroid cancer is a risk factor in both medullary and papillary thyroid cancer. The first-degree relatives could predict the risk of thyroid cancer [7]. A total of 10,709 participants was included in the study. Correlation of cytological findings and family history was evaluated using Fisher's exact test. There were 2580 (24.09%) patients with non-malignant thyroid diseases in the family and 198 (1.85%) patients with a history of thyroid cancer in the family. A total of 2778 (25.94%) patients had a positive family history of thyroid diseases, and 7931 (74.06%) patients had a negative family history. In patients with a family history of papillary thyroid carcinoma, the difference between those with benign and malignant thyroid tumors was found to be significant ($p = 0.0432$). Thyroid cancer may be more aggressive in younger patients and may have a higher rate of lymph node metastasis [7]. The rates for family histories of fathers and siblings were not different according to the age at onset of thyroid cancer, while those of mothers were higher in patients with a younger age at onset of thyroid cancer (Table 5). In addition, this study analyzed the interaction among familial histories by using the interaction model. There was no significant interactional effect in father with siblings and mother with siblings (Table 4).

Despite our large sample size, this study has few limitations. First, it was impossible to consider all the confounding factors for the association. KoGES did not cover all of the potentially influencing factors such as history of radiation therapy and CT, iodine intake, and history of thyroiditis. Second, KoGES HEXA was started based on a questionnaire survey [27]. The patient's thyroid cancer history was asked. However, in the cases of positivity, no biopsy or ultrasonography was performed for a definitive diagnosis. This study included all participants who had thyroid cancer as PTC given that about 95% of DTC cases in Korea were PTC [9]. Third, this study included only the participants who were survivors after being diagnosed with thyroid cancer. The survey could not be performed with the dead participants. However, this was not a huge problem because the survival rate of thyroid cancer in Korea is high. Thyroid cancer has an excellent prognosis and a five-year relative survival rate of 100.1% in Korea [43]. Lastly, this study did not include the family history of grandparents or distant relatives. Last, the reliability of the questionnaires on the smoking, alcohol consumption, and nutritional intake frequencies were unclear [27]. To collect accurate data, the reliability and validity of the questionnaire survey should be examined in future studies.

In contrast, this study has several advantages. To the best of our knowledge, this study is the first population-based study examining the association between thyroid cancer family history and the incidence of thyroid cancer in Asia. Second, this study is a large population-based study compared with studies in other countries. This study investigated detailed associations in subgroups in a large population. In addition, the risk of family history on incidence was evaluated using a large control group. This study provides more precise information than most previous individual studies. Third, this study considered many more influential factors than in previous studies. Obesity, smoking, and alcohol consumption were further adjusted in this study. These confounding factors would be important adjustments for the analysis of family history as a risk factor.

5. Conclusions

This study demonstrated that the incidence of thyroid cancer was associated with thyroid cancer family history. This finding supports regular examination of individuals with a family history of thyroid cancer to prevent the progression of thyroid cancer. The identification of family history would provide opportunities for early detection and prevention. Further studies including those on gene mutations associated with family history are recommended to demonstrate the pathophysiology and prevalence of thyroid cancer.

Author Contributions: Conceptualization, H.-G.C.; Data curation, C.M. and H.-G.C.; Formal analysis, C.M. and H.-G.C.; Funding acquisition, H.-G.C.; Investigation, S.-H.B. and H.-G.C.; Methodology, H.-G.C.; Project administration, S.-H.B. and H.-G.C.; Resources, S.-H.B.; Software, S.-J.H.; Supervision, S.-H.B. and S.-J.H.; Validation, S.-H.B.; Visualization, S.-J.H.; Writing—original draft, S.-H.B. and S.-J.H.; and Writing—review and editing, S.-H.B. and S.-J.H. All authors have read and agreed to the published version of the manuscript.

Funding: This work was supported in part by a research grant (NRF-2018-R1D1A1A0-2085328) from the National Research Foundation (NRF) of Korea and Hallym University Research Fund (HURF-2019-31). This study was supported by the National Research Foundation of Korea (NRF) grant funded by the Korean government Ministry of Science and ICT (No. 2017R1C1B5076558).

Conflicts of Interest: The authors declare no conflict of interest.

References

1. Vigneri, R.; Malandrino, P.; Vigneri, P. The changing epidemiology of thyroid cancer: Why is incidence increasing? *Curr. Opin. Oncol.* **2015**, *27*, 1–7. [CrossRef] [PubMed]
2. Morris, L.G.; Sikora, A.G.; Tosteson, T.D.; Davies, L. The increasing incidence of thyroid cancer: The influence of access to care. *Thyroid* **2013**, *23*, 885–891. [CrossRef] [PubMed]
3. Mazzaferri, E.L. Management of a solitary thyroid nodule. *N. Engl. J. Med.* **1993**, *328*, 553–559. [CrossRef] [PubMed]
4. Wartofsky, L. Increasing world incidence of thyroid cancer: Increased detection or higher radiation exposure? *Hormones* **2010**, *9*, 103–108. [CrossRef]
5. Ahn, H.S.; Kim, H.J.; Welch, H.G. Korea's thyroid-cancer "epidemic"—Screening and overdiagnosis. *N. Engl. J. Med.* **2014**, *371*, 1765–1767. [CrossRef]
6. Ferlay, J.; Colombet, M.; Soerjomataram, I.; Mathers, C.; Parkin, D.M.; Pineros, M.; Znaor, A.; Bray, F. Estimating the global cancer incidence and mortality in 2018: GLOBOCAN sources and methods. *Int. J. Cancer* **2019**, *144*, 1941–1953. [CrossRef]

7. Kust, D.; Stanicic, J.; Matesa, N. Bethesda thyroid categories and family history of thyroid disease. *Clin. Endocrinol.* **2018**, *88*, 468–472. [CrossRef]
8. Schmidbauer, B.; Menhart, K.; Hellwig, D.; Grosse, J. Differentiated Thyroid Cancer-Treatment: State of the Art. *Int. J. Mol. Sci.* **2017**, *18*, 1292. [CrossRef]
9. Park, S.; Oh, C.M.; Cho, H.; Lee, J.Y.; Jung, K.W.; Jun, J.K.; Won, Y.J.; Kong, H.J.; Choi, K.S.; Lee, Y.J.; et al. Association between screening and the thyroid cancer "epidemic" in South Korea: Evidence from a nationwide study. *BMJ* **2016**, *355*, i5745. [CrossRef]
10. Xing, M.; Haugen, B.R.; Schlumberger, M. Progress in molecular-based management of differentiated thyroid cancer. *Lancet* **2013**, *381*, 1058–1069. [CrossRef]
11. Spano, J.P.; Vano, Y.; Vignot, S.; De La Motte Rouge, T.; Hassani, L.; Mouawad, R.; Menegaux, F.; Khayat, D.; Leenhardt, L. GEMOX regimen in the treatment of metastatic differentiated refractory thyroid carcinoma. *Med. Oncol.* **2012**, *29*, 1421–1428. [CrossRef]
12. Crouzeix, G.; Michels, J.J.; Sevin, E.; Aide, N.; Vaur, D.; Bardet, S.; French, T.N. Unusual short-term complete response to two regimens of cytotoxic chemotherapy in a patient with poorly differentiated thyroid carcinoma. *J. Clin. Endocrinol. Metab.* **2012**, *97*, 3046–3050. [CrossRef]
13. Xu, L.; Li, G.; Wei, Q.; El-Naggar, A.K.; Sturgis, E.M. Family history of cancer and risk of sporadic differentiated thyroid carcinoma. *Cancer* **2012**, *118*, 1228–1235. [CrossRef]
14. Albi, E.; Cataldi, S.; Lazzarini, A.; Codini, M.; Beccari, T.; Ambesi-Impiombato, F.S.; Curcio, F. Radiation and Thyroid Cancer. *Int. J. Mol. Sci.* **2017**, *18*, 911. [CrossRef]
15. Pacini, F.; Castagna, M.G.; Brilli, L.; Pentheroudakis, G.; Group, E.G.W. Thyroid cancer: ESMO Clinical Practice Guidelines for diagnosis, treatment and follow-up. *Ann. Oncol.* **2012**, *23* (Suppl. 7), vii110–vii119. [CrossRef]
16. Cong, X. Air pollution from industrial waste gas emissions is associated with cancer incidences in Shanghai, China. *Environ. Sci. Pollut. Res. Int.* **2018**, *25*, 13067–13078. [CrossRef]
17. Fiore, M.; Oliveri Conti, G.; Caltabiano, R.; Buffone, A.; Zuccarello, P.; Cormaci, L.; Cannizzaro, M.A.; Ferrante, M. Role of Emerging Environmental Risk Factors in Thyroid Cancer: A Brief Review. *Int. J. Environ. Res. Public Health* **2019**, *16*, 1185. [CrossRef]
18. Mack, W.J.; Preston-Martin, S.; Dal Maso, L.; Galanti, R.; Xiang, M.; Franceschi, S.; Hallquist, A.; Jin, F.; Kolonel, L.; La Vecchia, C.; et al. A pooled analysis of case-control studies of thyroid cancer: Cigarette smoking and consumption of alcohol, coffee, and tea. *Cancer Causes Control.* **2003**, *14*, 773–785. [CrossRef]
19. Nikiforova, M.N.; Tseng, G.C.; Steward, D.; Diorio, D.; Nikiforov, Y.E. MicroRNA expression profiling of thyroid tumors: Biological significance and diagnostic utility. *J. Clin. Endocrinol. Metab.* **2008**, *93*, 1600–1608. [CrossRef]
20. Abdullah, M.I.; Junit, S.M.; Ng, K.L.; Jayapalan, J.J.; Karikalan, B.; Hashim, O.H. Papillary Thyroid Cancer: Genetic Alterations and Molecular Biomarker Investigations. *Int. J. Med. Sci.* **2019**, *16*, 450–460. [CrossRef]
21. Cooper, D.S.; Doherty, G.M.; Haugen, B.R.; Kloos, R.T.; Lee, S.L.; Mandel, S.J.; Mazzaferri, E.L.; McIver, B.; Pacini, F.; Schlumberger, M.; et al. Revised American Thyroid Association management guidelines for patients with thyroid nodules and differentiated thyroid cancer. *Thyroid* **2009**, *19*, 1167–1214. [CrossRef]
22. Fallah, M.; Sundquist, K.; Hemminki, K. Risk of thyroid cancer in relatives of patients with medullary thyroid carcinoma by age at diagnosis. *Endocr. Relat. Cancer* **2013**, *20*, 717–724. [CrossRef]
23. Goldgar, D.E.; Easton, D.F.; Cannon-Albright, L.A.; Skolnick, M.H. Systematic population-based assessment of cancer risk in first-degree relatives of cancer probands. *J. Natl. Cancer Inst.* **1994**, *86*, 1600–1608. [CrossRef]
24. Amundadottir, L.T.; Thorvaldsson, S.; Gudbjartsson, D.F.; Sulem, P.; Kristjansson, K.; Arnason, S.; Gulcher, J.R.; Bjornsson, J.; Kong, A.; Thorsteinsdottir, U.; et al. Cancer as a complex phenotype: Pattern of cancer distribution within and beyond the nuclear family. *PLoS Med.* **2004**, *1*, e65. [CrossRef]
25. Hwang, S.H.; Kim, E.K.; Moon, H.J.; Yoon, J.H.; Kwak, J.Y. Risk of Thyroid Cancer in Euthyroid Asymptomatic Patients with Thyroid Nodules with an Emphasis on Family History of Thyroid Cancer. *Korean J. Radiol.* **2016**, *17*, 255–263. [CrossRef]
26. Myung, S.K.; Lee, C.W.; Lee, J.; Kim, J.; Kim, H.S. Risk Factors for Thyroid Cancer: A Hospital-Based Case-Control Study in Korean Adults. *Cancer Res. Treat.* **2017**, *49*, 70–78. [CrossRef]
27. Byun, S.H.; Min, C.; Hong, S.J.; Choi, H.G.; Koh, D.H. Analysis of the Relation between Periodontitis and Chronic Gastritis/Peptic Ulcer: A Cross-Sectional Study Using KoGES HEXA Data. *Int. J. Environ. Res. Public Health* **2020**, *17*, 4387. [CrossRef]

28. Kim, Y.; Han, B.G.; KoGES Group. Cohort Profile: The Korean Genome and Epidemiology Study (KoGES) Consortium. *Int. J. Epidemiol.* **2017**, *46*, 1350. [CrossRef]
29. Byun, S.H.; Min, C.; Kim, Y.B.; Kim, H.; Kang, S.H.; Park, B.J.; Wee, J.H.; Choi, H.G.; Hong, S.J. Analysis of Chronic Periodontitis in Tonsillectomy Patients: A Longitudinal Follow-Up Study Using a National Health Screening Cohort. *Appl. Sci.* **2020**, *10*, 3663. [CrossRef]
30. Byun, S.H.; Min, C.; Park, I.S.; Kim, H.; Kim, S.K.; Park, B.J.; Choi, H.G.; Hong, S.J. Increased Risk of Chronic Periodontitis in Chronic Rhinosinusitis Patients: A Longitudinal Follow-Up Study Using a National Health-Screening Cohort. *J. Clin. Med.* **2020**, *9*, 1170. [CrossRef]
31. Byun, S.H.; Lee, S.; Kang, S.H.; Choi, H.G.; Hong, S.J. Cross-Sectional Analysis of the Association between Periodontitis and Cardiovascular Disease Using the Korean Genome and Epidemiology Study Data. *Int. J. Environ. Res. Public Health* **2020**, *17*, 5237. [CrossRef]
32. Tavarelli, M.; Russo, M.; Terranova, R.; Scollo, C.; Spadaro, A.; Sapuppo, G.; Malandrino, P.; Masucci, R.; Squatrito, S.; Pellegriti, G. Familial Non-Medullary Thyroid Cancer Represents an Independent Risk Factor for Increased Cancer Aggressiveness: A Retrospective Analysis of 74 Families. *Front. Endocrinol.* **2015**, *6*, 117. [CrossRef]
33. Oakley, G.M.; Curtin, K.; Pimentel, R.; Buchmann, L.; Hunt, J. Establishing a familial basis for papillary thyroid carcinoma using the Utah Population Database. *JAMA Otolaryngol. Head Neck Surg.* **2013**, *139*, 1171–1174. [CrossRef]
34. Ahn, H.S.; Kim, H.J.; Kim, K.H.; Lee, Y.S.; Han, S.J.; Kim, Y.; Ko, M.J.; Brito, J.P. Thyroid Cancer Screening in South Korea Increases Detection of Papillary Cancers with No Impact on Other Subtypes or Thyroid Cancer Mortality. *Thyroid* **2016**, *26*, 1535–1540. [CrossRef]
35. Brito, J.P.; Kim, H.J.; Han, S.J.; Lee, Y.S.; Ahn, H.S. Geographic Distribution and Evolution of Thyroid Cancer Epidemic in South Korea. *Thyroid* **2016**, *26*, 864–865. [CrossRef]
36. Oh, C.M.; Kong, H.J.; Kim, E.; Kim, H.; Jung, K.W.; Park, S.; Won, Y.J. National Epidemiologic Survey of Thyroid cancer (NEST) in Korea. *Epidemiol. Health* **2018**, *40*, e2018052. [CrossRef]
37. Zhao, Z.G.; Guo, X.G.; Ba, C.X.; Wang, W.; Yang, Y.Y.; Wang, J.; Cao, H.Y. Overweight, obesity and thyroid cancer risk: A meta-analysis of cohort studies. *J. Int. Med. Res.* **2012**, *40*, 2041–2050. [CrossRef]
38. Han, J.M.; Kim, T.Y.; Jeon, M.J.; Yim, J.H.; Kim, W.G.; Song, D.E.; Hong, S.J.; Bae, S.J.; Kim, H.K.; Shin, M.H.; et al. Obesity is a risk factor for thyroid cancer in a large, ultrasonographically screened population. *Eur. J. Endocrinol.* **2013**, *168*, 879–886. [CrossRef]
39. Cho, Y.A.; Kim, J. Thyroid cancer risk and smoking status: A meta-analysis. *Cancer Causes Control.* **2014**, *25*, 1187–1195. [CrossRef]
40. Kitahara, C.M.; Linet, M.S.; Beane Freeman, L.E.; Check, D.P.; Church, T.R.; Park, Y.; Purdue, M.P.; Schairer, C.; Berrington de Gonzalez, A. Cigarette smoking, alcohol intake, and thyroid cancer risk: A pooled analysis of five prospective studies in the United States. *Cancer Causes Control.* **2012**, *23*, 1615–1624. [CrossRef]
41. Balhara, Y.P.; Deb, K.S. Impact of alcohol use on thyroid function. *Indian J. Endocrinol. Metab.* **2013**, *17*, 580–587. [CrossRef]
42. Hong, S.H.; Myung, S.K.; Kim, H.S.; Korean Meta-Analysis Study, G. Alcohol Intake and Risk of Thyroid Cancer: A Meta-Analysis of Observational Studies. *Cancer Res. Treat.* **2017**, *49*, 534–547. [CrossRef]
43. Hong, S.; Won, Y.J.; Park, Y.R.; Jung, K.W.; Kong, H.J.; Lee, E.S.; The Community of Population-Based Regional Cancer Registries. Cancer Statistics in Korea: Incidence, Mortality, Survival, and Prevalence in 2017. *Cancer Res. Treat.* **2020**, *52*, 335–350. [CrossRef]

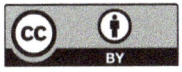

© 2020 by the authors. Licensee MDPI, Basel, Switzerland. This article is an open access article distributed under the terms and conditions of the Creative Commons Attribution (CC BY) license (http://creativecommons.org/licenses/by/4.0/).

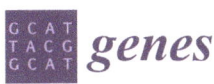

Article

Micronuclei Formation upon Radioiodine Therapy for Well-Differentiated Thyroid Cancer: The Influence of DNA Repair Genes Variants

Luís S. Santos [1,2], Octávia M. Gil [3], Susana N. Silva [1,*], Bruno C. Gomes [1], Teresa C. Ferreira [4], Edward Limbert [5] and José Rueff [1]

[1] Centre for Toxicogenomics and Human Health (ToxOmics), Genetics, Oncology and Human Toxicology, NOVA Medical School; Faculdade de Ciências Médicas, Universidade Nova de Lisboa, 1169-056 Lisboa, Portugal; lsilvasantos@gmail.com (L.S.S.); bruno.gomes@nms.unl.pt (B.C.G.); jose.rueff@nms.unl.pt (J.R.)
[2] Institute of Health Sciences (ICS), Center for Interdisciplinary Research in Health (CIIS), Universidade Católica Portuguesa, 3504-505 Viseu, Portugal
[3] Centro de Ciências e Tecnologias Nucleares, Instituto Superior Técnico, Universidade de Lisboa, 2695-066 Bobadela, Loures, Portugal; ogil@ctn.tecnico.ulisboa.pt
[4] Serviço de Medicina Nuclear, Instituto Português de Oncologia de Lisboa (IPOLFG), 1099-023 Lisboa, Portugal; teresa.ferreira_medical@yahoo.com
[5] Serviço de Endocrinologia, Instituto Português de Oncologia de Lisboa (IPOLFG), 1099-023 Lisboa, Portugal; elimbert@ipolisboa.min-saude.pt
* Correspondence: snsilva@nms.unl.pt

Received: 4 August 2020; Accepted: 15 September 2020; Published: 17 September 2020

Abstract: Radioiodine therapy with ^{131}I remains the mainstay of standard treatment for well-differentiated thyroid cancer (DTC). Prognosis is good but concern exists that ^{131}I-emitted ionizing radiation may induce double-strand breaks in extra-thyroidal tissues, increasing the risk of secondary malignancies. We, therefore, sought to evaluate the induction and 2-year persistence of micronuclei (MN) in lymphocytes from 26 ^{131}I-treated DTC patients and the potential impact of nine homologous recombination (HR), non-homologous end-joining (NHEJ), and mismatch repair (MMR) polymorphisms on MN levels. MN frequency was determined by the cytokinesis-blocked micronucleus assay while genotyping was performed through pre-designed TaqMan® Assays or conventional PCR-restriction fragment length polymorphism (RFLP). MN levels increased significantly one month after therapy and remained persistently higher than baseline for 2 years. A marked reduction in lymphocyte proliferation capacity was also apparent 2 years after therapy. *MLH1* rs1799977 was associated with MN frequency (absolute or net variation) one month after therapy, in two independent groups. Significant associations were also observed for *MSH3* rs26279, *MSH4* rs5745325, *NBN* rs1805794, and tumor histotype. Overall, our results suggest that ^{131}I therapy may pose a long-term challenge to cells other than thyrocytes and that the individual genetic profile may influence ^{131}I sensitivity, hence its risk-benefit ratio. Further studies are warranted to confirm the potential utility of these single nucleotide polymorphisms (SNPs) as radiogenomic biomarkers in the personalization of radioiodine therapy.

Keywords: thyroid cancer; Iodine-131; chromosome-defective micronuclei; DNA repair; micronucleus assay; single nucleotide polymorphism; pharmacogenomic variants; pharmacogenetics; precision medicine

1. Introduction

Thyroid cancer (TC) is the most common endocrine malignancy, accounting for approximately 2.1% of cancers diagnosed all over the world. TC incidence is about two to four times higher in women than in men and is one of the most common malignancies in adolescent and young adults (ages 15–39 years), with the median age at diagnosis being lower than that for most other types of cancer [1–3]. TC incidence has been steadily increasing, over the last three decades [1], most likely because of "surveillance bias" and overdiagnosis resulting from increased detection of small stationary lesions of limited clinical relevance. A true rise in the number of TC cases (e.g., due to increasing exposure to ionizing radiation (IR) from medical sources) is, however, also possible [2–4].

Papillary (PTC) and follicular (FTC) thyroid carcinoma represent 85–90% and 5–10% of TC cases, respectively. These tumor histotypes retain their morphologic features, being often referred to as differentiated thyroid carcinoma (DTC) [3,4]. The best-established modifiable risk factor for DTC is IR exposure during childhood and adolescence (radioiodines including ^{131}I, X-radiation, γ-radiation) [2–5] and the standard treatment consists of surgical resection (total or near-total thyroidectomy) accompanied by post-thyroidectomy radioiodine (RAI) therapy and TSH suppression [3,4]. The majority of DTC cases is indolent in nature, iodine-avid, and responds favorably to standard therapy. Overall prognosis is thus generally good, translating into high long-term survival and low disease-specific mortality [4].

The widespread use of RAI therapy in the management of DTC relies on the ability of ^{131}I to be preferentially taken up and concentrated in normal or neoplastic thyroid follicular cells, taking advantage of these cells' specialized mechanism for iodide uptake and accumulation [3,6,7]. Thyrocyte-accumulated ^{131}I undergoes [β and γ] decay and releases high-energy electrons that inflict devastating DNA damage locally. Thyroid cell death through radiation cytotoxicity ensues, allowing for the ablation of remnant normal thyroid tissue and the eradication of any residual tumor foci [3,6]. Unfortunately, since other tissues may also concentrate ^{131}I, its DNA damaging effects may not be limited to the thyroid gland, increasing the risk of RAI-associated secondary malignancies such as soft tissue tumors, colorectal cancer, salivary tumors, and leukemia [3,7]. Since the rising incidence of TC is mostly driven by increased detection of stationary subclinical lesions, concern exists that DTC overdiagnosis may result in potentially harmful overtreatment [2]. Indeed, if we consider the indolent behavior of the disease, its long-term survival rate, and its mean age of diagnosis, such therapy-related morbidity may not be justified, as most patients will have many years to experience its negative effects [2]. The revised American Thyroid Association (ATA) clinical practice guidelines for the management of DTC [8] reflect such concern for the first time, recommending a more cautious diagnosis and treatment approach in order to reduce RAI use (hence, radiation exposure) particularly in younger ages. This includes, for example, more stringent criteria for diagnosis upon nodule detection, molecular-based risk stratification for improved treatment decisions, personalized disease management and long-term surveillance strategies and, most importantly, use of lower RAI doses (30–50 mCi) in patients with low-risk DTC [2,8,9].

The most relevant types of DNA damage inflicted upon IR exposure are double-strand breaks (DSBs). Such lesions are predominantly processed by DNA repair enzymes of the homologous recombination (HR) and non-homologous end-joining (NHEJ) repair pathways, despite mismatch repair (MMR) pathway enzymes have also been implicated [10,11]. The activity of such DNA repair enzymes determines the capacity of cells to repair DSBs which, in turn, influences their sensitivity to IR. Lower DNA repair capacity, therefore, increases the extent of IR-induced DNA damage, increasing both the likelihood of cell death through IR-induced cytotoxicity and the likelihood of malignant transformation upon IR exposure [12,13].

Single nucleotide polymorphisms (SNPs) in DNA repair enzymes across these three pathways have been identified and some have been demonstrated to affect the DNA repair capacity [14,15]. Such DNA repair SNPs may therefore modulate sensitivity to IR and many have indeed been associated with TC or, more specifically, DTC susceptibility (for which IR exposure is the best-established risk factor) [16–21]. It is likely that such functional DNA repair SNPs, through interference with the extent of IR-induced DSBs on thyrocytes, could influence the cytotoxic potential of RAI therapy, hence its efficacy on DTC treatment. Likewise, through a similar effect on other cells that take up and concentrate ^{131}I, such SNPs could also modify the risk of secondary malignancies, hence the safety of RAI therapy.

Identifying these variants is, therefore, an important challenge with clinical relevance. However, to our knowledge, the issue has not been addressed in prior studies.

We have previously demonstrated that therapy with 70 mCi ^{131}I in DTC patients is consistently associated with increased DNA damage levels in peripheral lymphocytes [22,23]. With this study, we aimed to confirm, through the use of the cytokinesis-blocked micronucleus (CBMN) assay, our prior findings in a new group of DTC patients submitted to RAI therapy with 100 mCi. Further, we sought to extend our analysis at 24 months after ^{131}I administration so that the long-term persistence of ^{131}I-induced DNA damage could be better characterized. Finally, the potential influence of HR, NHEJ, and MMR polymorphisms on the micronuclei (MN) frequency in RAI-treated DTC patients was also investigated.

Understanding the role of repair SNPs on the extent and persistence of ^{131}I-induced DNA damage will contribute to the identification of genetic biomarkers that influence the individual response to ^{131}I-based RAI therapy and thus modulate the risk-benefit ratio of RAI therapy in DTC patients. Such efforts may provide the basis for improved, personalized, therapeutic decisions in the context of DTC therapy, with impact on disease prognosis and patient safety.

2. Materials and Methods

2.1. Study Population

Twenty-six DTC patients proposed for radioiodine therapy at the Department of Nuclear Medicine of the Portuguese Oncology Institute of Lisbon (Portugal) were selected according to criteria published elsewhere [22]. All participants were treated according to current practice, consisting of total thyroidectomy followed by oral administration of ^{131}I, 70 mCi (15 patients) or 100 mCi (11 patients), to ablate thyroid remnant cells. Patients were followed for two years unless they had to be submitted to further treatment. In such cases, patients were no longer elective for cytogenetic analysis and had to be excluded from further analysis. A mixed cross-sectional and longitudinal study design was used, respectively, for comparisons among genotypes or dose groups at each time point and across different time points. In the latter case, pre-treatment values allowed each patient to serve as his own control.

To characterize the study population and account for potential confounding factors, all participants were interviewed and completed a detailed questionnaire covering standard demographic characteristics, personal and family medical history, lifestyle habits, and prior IR exposure. For the purpose of smoking status, former smokers who had quit smoking at least 2 years prior to diagnosis were considered as non-smokers. Clinical and pathological examination was also performed.

Peripheral blood samples were collected from each patient into both 10 mL heparinized tubes (for cytogenetic analysis) and citrated tubes (for genotype analysis). For cytogenetic analysis, blood samples were drawn (1) prior to ^{131}I administration as well as 1, 6, and 24 months after therapy in patients submitted to a 70 mCi dose and (2) prior to ^{131}I administration as well as 1 and 3 months afterward in patients submitted to a 100 mCi dose. For genotype analysis, blood samples were stored at −80 °C until further use.

All subjects gave their informed consent for inclusion before they participated in the study. The study was conducted in accordance with the Declaration of Helsinki, and the protocol was approved by the Ethics Committee of Instituto Português de Oncologia Francisco Gentil (GIC/357) and by the Ethics Committee of Faculdade Ciências Médicas (CE-5/2008).

2.2. Genotype Analysis

Genomic DNA was isolated from blood samples using the commercially available QIAamp® DNA mini kit (QIAamp® DNA mini kit; Qiagen GmbH, Hilden, Germany), according to the manufacturer's recommendations. The fluorimetric Quant-iT™ Picogreen® dsDNA Assay Kit (Invitrogen, Waltham, MA, USA) was used to quantify and ensure uniformity in DNA concentration (2.5 ng/µL). DNA samples were kept at −20 °C until further use.

SNPs were selected from those already analyzed by our team in a cohort of 106 DTC patients, according to selection criteria published elsewhere [18–21]. Due to sample size limitations, only SNPs presenting a minor allele frequency (MAF) > 0.15 in the original pool of patients were considered. *MLH3* rs175080 was excluded *a posteriori* for insufficient genotype frequency ($n \leq 1$) in at least one of the ^{131}I dose groups (Table S1). Overall, a total of 9 DNA repair SNPs across 3 DNA repair pathways (HR, NHEJ, and MMR) were considered for further analysis (Table 1).

Table 1. Selected SNPs and detailed information on the corresponding base and amino acid changes, minor allele frequency, and Applied Biosystems (AB) assay used for genotyping.

Gene	Location	DB SNP Cluster ID (RS NO.)	Base Change	Amino Acid Change	MAF (%) [a]	AB Assay ID
MLH1	3p22.2	rs1799977	A → G	Ile219Val	23.3	C___1219076_20
MSH3	5q14.1	rs26279	A → G	Thr1045Ala	27.1	C___800002_1_
MSH4	1p31.1	rs5745325	G → A	Ala97Thr	26.0	C___3286081_10
PMS1	2q32.2	rs5742933	G → C	– [b]	23.4	C___29329633_10
MSH6	2p16.3	rs1042821	C → T	Gly39Glu	18.2	C___8760558_10
RAD51	15q15.1	rs1801321	G → T	– [b]	33.2	C___7482700_10
NBN	8q21.3	rs1805794	G → C	Glu185Gln	34.7	C___26470398_30
XRCC3	14q32.33	rs861539	C → T	Thr241Met	29.0	– [d]
XRCC5	2q35	rs2440	C → T	– [c]	36.3	C___3231046_10

[a] MAF, minor allele frequency, according to the Genome Aggregation Database (gnomAD), v2.1.1, available at https://gnomad.broadinstitute.org/. [b] SNP located on 5' UTR. [c] SNP located on 3' UTR. [d] not applicable (genotyping performed by PCR-RFLP). SNPs, single nucleotide polymorphisms.

Genotyping was performed mostly by real-time polymerase chain reaction (RT-PCR): amplification and allelic discrimination were carried out on a 96-well ABI 7300 Real-Time PCR system thermal cycler (Applied Biosystems; Thermo Fisher Scientific, Inc., Waltham, MA, USA), following the manufacturer's instructions, with the use of the commercially available TaqMan® SNP Genotyping Assays (Applied Biosystems) identified in Table 1. For *XRCC3* rs861539 (HR pathway), genotyping was performed by conventional PCR-restriction fragment length polymorphism (RFLP) techniques. Primer sequences, PCR, and digestion conditions as well as expected electrophoretic patterns have been described [19]. To confirm genotyping and ensure accurate results, inconclusive samples were reanalyzed and genotyping was repeated in 10–15% of randomly chosen samples, with 100% concordance.

2.3. Cytogenetic Analysis

The cytokinesis-block micronucleus assay (CBMN) was used to analyze DNA damage and conducted according to standard methods. The methodology was performed and published as described previously [22–24]. The frequency of binucleated cells carrying micronuclei (BNMN), defined as the number of cells with MN per 1000 binucleated lymphocytes, is expressed as a count per thousand (‰). The Cytokinesis-Block Proliferation Index (CBPI) was determined according to the formula CBPI = [MI + 2MII + 3(MIII + MIV)]/N, where MI-MIV correspond to the number of human lymphocytes with one to four nuclei, respectively, and N is the total number of cells analyzed.

2.4. Statistical Analysis

All analyses were done with SPSS 22.0 (IBM SPSS Statistics for Windows, version 22.0, IBM Corp, Armonk, NY, USA) except for deviation of genotype distributions from Hardy–Weinberg equilibrium (HWE) and linkage disequilibrium (LD) analysis between SNPs on the same chromosome, which were performed with SNPstats [25].

Categorical variables, presented as frequencies and percentages, were compared between dose groups and with the original cohort of DTC patients by the Pearson's Chi-square (χ^2) test or the two-sided Fisher's exact test whenever 2 × 2 contingency tables were possible. For continuous variables (BNMN frequency, CBPI, and their net variation from baseline), presented as mean ± standard deviation, the normality and homogeneity of variances were evaluated by the Shapiro-Wilk and Levene tests, respectively. Longitudinal comparisons were performed by the paired sample t test (whenever a normal distribution could not be excluded) or the Wilcoxon signed-rank test (remaining cases) while the parametric Student t test (normal distributions) or the nonparametric Mann-Whitney U test (non-normal distributions) for independent samples were used for cross-sectional comparisons between the two ^{131}I dose groups and between different gender, age class, smoking status, histological type of tumor, and genotype categories.

Variable transformation was considered, when practically useful: DTC patients were dichotomized according to age, with the cut-off point being defined as the median age of all patients included (54 years). Due to limited sample size (hence, low frequency of homozygous variant genotypes), a dominant model of inheritance was assumed for all SNPs. Moreover, the net variation in BNMN frequency (i.e., therapy-induced BNMN) was calculated by subtracting the background (pre-treatment) BNMN frequency from the corresponding post-treatment values.

This is an exploratory 'proof of concept' study, not a conclusive final one. As such, the Bonferroni adjustment was deemed as not necessary as it is too conservative. Furthermore, the complement of the false-negative rate β to compute the power of a test (1-β) was not taken into account at this stage since larger studies are needed to change this preliminary study into a confirmatory one. Statistical significance was set at $p < 0.05$.

3. Results

3.1. Characteristics of the Study Population

A general description of the study population is presented in Table 2. The age of DTC patients submitted to ^{131}I therapy ranged from 32 to 73 years, with a mean of 52.54 ± 11.62 years. As expected, female patients (88.5%, $n = 23$) greatly outnumbered male patients (11.5%, $n = 3$) and papillary carcinoma cases (PTC, 69.2%, $n = 18$) were also more frequent than follicular ones (FTC, 30.8%, $n = 8$), in agreement with gender and histotype distributions commonly reported for DTC [1,2,4]. Overall, 15.4% ($n = 4$) of patients were smokers. No significant differences in patient age, gender, histological type of tumor, and smoking status were observed between groups submitted to different ^{131}I doses (Table 2) nor between any of these groups (separated or together) and our original DTC population [18].

Table 2. General characteristics for differentiated thyroid carcinoma (DTC) patients treated with 70 mCi ($n = 15$) and 100 mCi ($n = 11$) ^{131}I.

Characteristics	Study Population n (%)	70 mCi n (%)	100 mCi n (%)	p Value [c]
Gender				
Male	3 (11.5)	1 (6.7)	2 (18.2)	0.556
Female	23 (88.5)	14 (93.3)	9 (81.8)	
Age [a]	52.54 ± 11.62 [b]	52.07 ± 10.26 [b]	53.18 ± 13.76 [b]	0.815
≤54	14 (53.8)	8 (53.3)	6 (54.5)	1.000
>54	12 (46.2)	7 (46.7)	5 (45.5)	
Smoking habits				
Non-smokers	22 (84.6)	13 (86.7)	9 (81.8)	1.000
Smokers	4 (15.4)	2 (13.3)	2 (18.2)	
Histology				
Papillary	18 (69.2)	10 (66.7)	8 (72.7)	1.000
Follicular	8 (30.8)	5 (33.3)	3 (27.3)	

[a] For age categorization purposes, the median age of all patients included in the study (54 years) was defined as the cut-off point. [b] mean ± S.D. [c] p value for 70 mCi versus 100 mCi groups determined by two-sided Fisher's exact test (gender, smoking habits, and age categories) or Student t test (age mean ± S.D.).

3.2. Cytogenetic Data

The frequency of BNMN (mean ± S.D.) in the 26 DTC patients submitted to ^{131}I therapy and included in this study is illustrated in Figure 1 and summarized in Table S2. Pre-treatment and post-treatment values are presented, stratified by dose group.

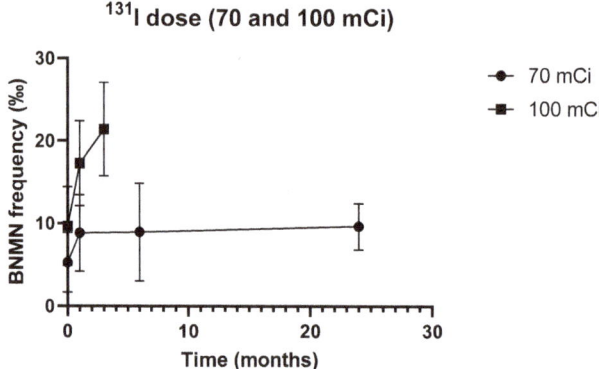

Figure 1. Binucleated cells carrying micronuclei (BNMN) frequency (‰, mean ± S.D.) in DTC patients before and after (1, 3/6, and 24 months) therapy with different doses of ^{131}I (70 and 100 mCi).

The results from the 70 mCi dose group until 6 months after ^{131}I administration have been published before [22]. As it was not possible to collect genotyping data on 4 of the original 19 patients, these patients were excluded and the data were re-analyzed. Longitudinal results in this dose group are, nevertheless, similar to those originally reported [22]: as evident from Figure 1, BNMN frequency in these patients increases significantly 1 month after ^{131}I therapy (from 5.27 ± 3.63‰ to 8.80 ± 4.65‰, $p = 0.039$) and stabilizes at 6 months after ^{131}I therapy (8.93 ± 5.92‰, $p = 0.944$ vs. 1 month after therapy), remaining persistently higher than before treatment ($p = 0.041$).

To investigate the long-term persistence of such therapy-induced damage, the study of these patients at 2 years after therapy was extended (Table S2 and Figure 1). Cytogenetic data at such time point was available for 11 patients only. The frequency of BNMN remained stable (9.64 ± 2.80‰, similar to values at 1 and 6 months, $p = 0.460$ and $p = 0.328$, respectively) and persistently higher than baseline ($p = 0.005$).

To confirm these findings and check for a possible dose effect, the study was replicated in an independent group of patients administered with 100 mCi. As expected, BNMN frequency was significantly higher in the 100 mCi group than in the 70 mCi group, irrespective of the time point (Table S2 and Figure 1), suggesting a dose-effect association (hence, a cause-effect relation) between iodine dose and BNMN levels. Apart from this quantitative difference, the effect of either dose on BNMN frequency was qualitatively similar, BNMN in the 100 mCi group increasing significantly 1 month after therapy (from 9.64 ± 4.78‰ to 17.27 ± 5.14‰, $p = 0.011$) and remaining persistently higher than baseline at 3 months (21.40 ± 5.66‰, $p < 0.001$ and $p = 0.054$ compared to pre-treatment and 1 month post-treatment values, respectively) (Table S2).

Moreover, of notice, the BNMN increment (net balance) after ^{131}I therapy was more pronounced in the 100 mCi group than in the 70 mCi group, despite the difference was not significant ($p > 0.05$).

Finally, the CBPI (mean ± S.D.) was also determined for the 15 DTC patients submitted to therapy with 70 mCi ^{131}I. As depicted in Figure 2, this index, which indicates the proliferation capacity of lymphocytes and may be used to calculate cytotoxicity [26], did not change appreciably at 1 and 6 months after ^{131}I administration but was markedly reduced at 24 months after therapy (from 1.78 ± 0.13 to 1.53 ± 0.09, $p = 0.001$).

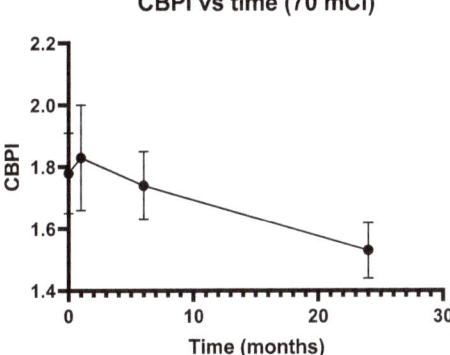

Figure 2. Cytokinesis-Block Proliferation Index (CBPI) (mean ± S.D.) in DTC patients before and after (1, 6, and 24 months) therapy with ^{131}I (70 mCi).

3.3. Characteristics of the Study Population and Cytogenetic Data

The potential influence of the demographic, lifestyle, and clinical characteristics of the study population on cytogenetic data was also evaluated. As depicted in Figure 3, in patients treated with 70 mCi, histology interfered with both pre-treatment BNMN levels and its net balance 1 month after ^{131}I therapy (Figure 3): basal BNMN frequency was significantly higher in FTC than in PTC patients (8.20 ± 3.11‰ vs. 3.80 ± 3.01‰, $p = 0.020$) but, 1 month after therapy, increased only in PTC patients, resulting in a significantly different net balance between the two histotypes (+6.20 ± 5.05‰ in PTC vs. −1.80 ± 3.96‰ in FTC, $p = 0.009$). Such effect was not observed in 100 mCi-treated patients nor when both dose groups were considered together. Likewise, no significant effect of gender, age, or smoking habits on BNMN levels or its net balance was detected, irrespective of the time point or dose group. Furthermore, except maybe for gender, no significant effect on CBPI was observed for any of these variables in the 70 mCi dose group. Baseline CBPI values were borderline higher in female compared to male patients ($p = 0.045$) but such finding should not be overvalued as only one male patient was included in this dose group.

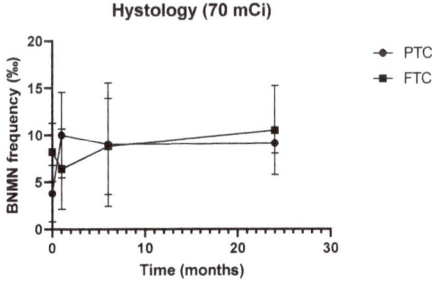

Figure 3. BNMN frequency (‰, mean ± S.D.) in DTC patients before and after (1, 6, and 24 months) therapy with 70 mCi ^{131}I, according to tumor histotype (papillary thyroid carcinoma (PTC) and follicular thyroid carcinoma (FTC)).

3.4. Distribution of DNA Repair SNPs in the Study Population

Table 3 reports the allele frequency and genotype distribution of 9 DNA repair SNPs among our sample of ^{131}I-treated patients. Genotype distributions were consistent with HWE in either dose group or their combination ($p > 0.05$) and, except for *MSH3* rs26279, did not differ significantly from those described in our previously studied DTC population ([c]). For *MSH3* rs26279, non-uniform distribution was observed, with the common allele being overrepresented in the study sample compared to the original population ($p = 0.048$, in the dominant model, Table S1). Moreover, importantly, no significant differences in genotype distributions were detected between dose groups, for any of the SNPs, irrespective of the model of inheritance assumed (Table 3). No relevant linkage association was observed between any of the SNPs.

Table 3. Allele and genotype frequencies in DTC patients submitted to ^{131}I therapy.

Genotype	70 mCi (n = 15)		100 mCi (n = 11)		TOTAL (n = 26)	
	MAF	Genotype Frequency n (%)	MAF	Genotype Frequency n (%)	MAF	Genotype Frequency n (%)
MLH1 rs1799977						
Ile/Ile		7 (46.7)		3 (27.3)		10 (38.5)
Ile/Val	G: 0.30	7 (46.7)	G: 0.45	6 (54.5)	G: 0.37	13 (50.0)
Val/Val		1 (6.7)		2 (18.2)		3 (11.5)
Ile/Val+Val/Val		8 (53.3)		8 (72.7)		16 (61.5)
MSH3 rs26279						
Thr/Thr		10 (66.7)		8 (72.7)		18 (69.2)
Thr/Ala	G: 0.23	3 (20.0)	G: 0.14	3 (27.3)	G: 0.19	6 (23.1)
Ala/Ala		2 (13.3)		0 (0.0)		2 (7.7)
Thr/Ala+Ala/Ala		5 (33.3)		3 (27.3)		8 (30.8)
MSH4 rs5745325						
Ala/Ala		11 (73.3)		4 (36.4)		15 (57.7)
Ala/Thr	A: 0.13	4 (26.7)	A: 0.32	7 (63.6)	A: 0.21	11 (42.3)
Thr/Thr		0 (0.0)		0 (0.0)		0 (0.0)
Ala/Thr+Thr/Thr		4 (26.7)		7 (63.6)		11 (42.3)
PMS1 rs5742933						
G/G		10 (71.4)		9 (81.8)		19 (76.0)
G/C	C: 0.18	3 (21.4)	C: 0.14	1 (9.1)	C: 0.16	4 (16.0)
C/C		1 (7.1)		1 (9.1)		2 (8.0)
G/C+C/C		4 (28.6)		2 (18.2)		6 (24.0)
MSH6 rs1042821						
Gly/Gly		10 (66.7)		9 (81.8)		19 (73.1)
Gly/Glu	T: 0.17	5 (33.3)	T: 0.09	2 (18.2)	T: 0.13	7 (26.9)
Glu/Glu		0 (0.0)		0 (0.0)		0 (0.0)
Gly/Glu+Glu/Glu		5 (33.3)		2 (18.2)		7 (26.9)
RAD51 rs1801321						
T/T		4 (26.7)		4 (36.4)		8 (30.8)
T/G	G: 0.50	7 (46.7)	G: 0.45	4 (36.4)	G: 0.48	11 (42.3)
G/G		4 (26.7)		3 (27.3)		7 (26.9)
T/G+G/G		11 (73.3)		7 (63.6)		18 (69.2)
NBN rs1805794						
Glu/Glu		7 (46.7)		8 (72.7)		15 (57.7)
Glu/Gln	C: 0.30	7 (46.7)	C: 0.14	3 (27.3)	C: 0.23	10 (38.5)
Gln/Gln		1 (6.7)		0 (0.0)		1 (3.8)
Glu/Gln+Gln/Gln		8 (53.3)		3 (27.3)		11 (42.3)
XRCC3 rs861539						
Thr/Thr		5 (33.3)		5 (45.5)		10 (38.5)
Thr/Met	C: 0.47	4 (26.7)	T: 0.36	4 (36.4)	T: 0.46	8 (30.8)
Met/Met		6 (40.0)		2 (18.2)		8 (30.8)
Thr/Met+Met/Met		10 (66.7)		6 (54.5)		16 (61.5)
XRCC5 rs2440						
T/T		5 (33.3)		2 (22.2)		7 (29.2)
T/C	C: 0.47	6 (40.0)	C: 0.50	5 (55.6)	C: 0.48	11 (45.8)
C/C		4 (26.7)		2 (22.2)		6 (25.0)
T/C+C/C		10 (66.7)		7 (77.8)		17 (70.8)

MAF, minor allele frequency. All comparisons of genotype distributions were performed by the two-sided Fisher's exact test (whenever 2 × 2 contingency tables are possible) or the χ^2 test (remaining cases). No significant differences among the 70 and 100 mCi dose groups were observed.

3.5. DNA Repair SNPs and Cytogenetic Data

The influence of DNA repair SNPs on BNMN frequencies and the corresponding variation from pre-treatment values is shown in Figure 4, Table 4, Table 5 and Tables S3–S5.

Prior to ^{131}I administration, BNMN frequency was higher in patients carrying the *MLH1* rs1799977 variant allele than in those homozygous for the common allele, with the difference being significant in the 100 mCi dose group ($p = 0.012$) and in the pool of both groups ($p = 0.019$).

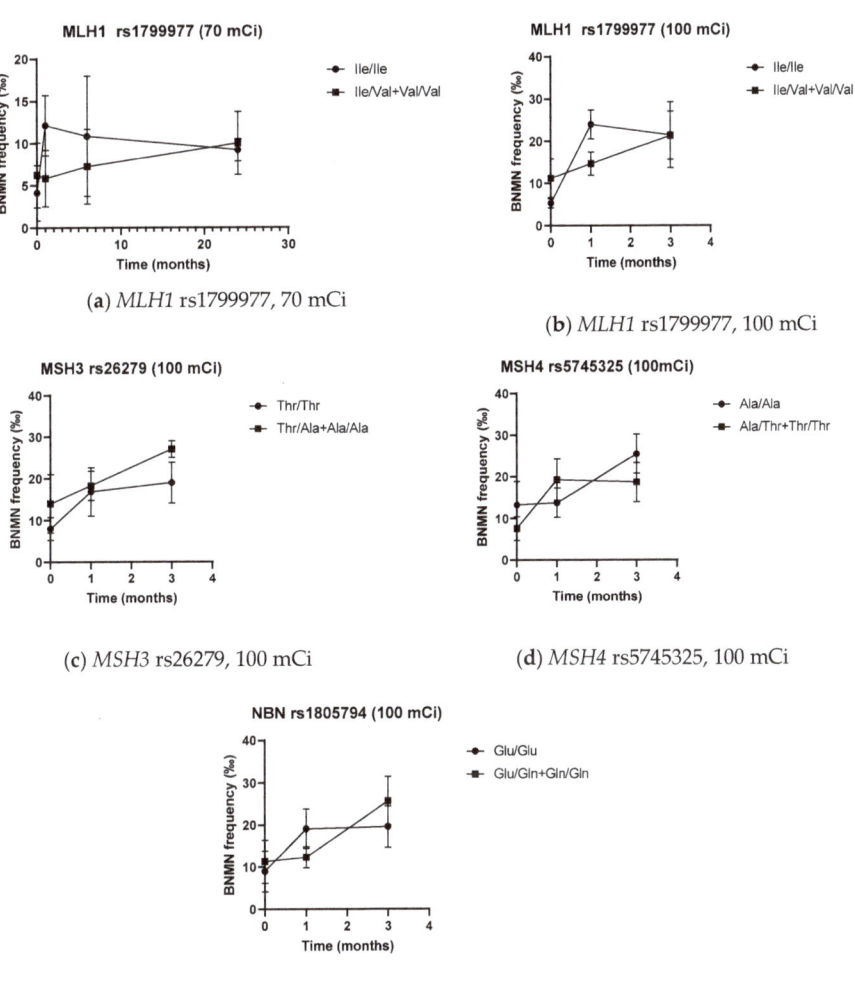

(a) *MLH1* rs1799977, 70 mCi

(b) *MLH1* rs1799977, 100 mCi

(c) *MSH3* rs26279, 100 mCi

(d) *MSH4* rs5745325, 100 mCi

(e) *NBN* rs1805794, 100 mCi

Figure 4. BNMN frequency (‰, mean ± S.D.) in DTC patients before and after (1, 3/6, and 24 months) therapy with ^{131}I, according to genotype and ^{131}I dose group: (**a**) *MLH1* rs1799977, 70 mCi; (**b**) *MLH1* rs1799977, 100 mCi; (**c**) *MSH3* rs26279, 100 mCi; (**d**) *MSH4* rs5745325, 100 mCi; (**e**) *NBN* rs1805794, 100 mCi.

Table 4. Frequency of micronucleated cells (‰BNMN, mean ± SD) in each ^{131}I dose group at t_0, t_1, t_3/t_6, and t_{24}, according to genotype (only SNP's presenting significant findings are shown).

Genotype	70 mCi Group (n = 15), ‰BNMN (Mean ± SD)				100 mCi Group (n = 11), ‰BNMN (Mean ± SD)			70 + 100 mCi Groups (n = 26), ‰BNMN (Mean ± SD)	
	t_0	t_1	t_6	t_{24}	t_0	t_1	t_3	t_0	t_1
MLH1 rs1799977									
Ile/Ile	4.14 ± 3.29	12.14 ± 3.58	10.86 ± 7.11	9.20 ± 1.30	5.33 ± 1.16	24.00 ± 3.46	21.50 ± 7.78	4.50 ± 2.80	15.70 ± 6.63
Ile/Val + Val/Val	6.25 ± 3.85	**5.88 ± 3.36 ***	7.25 ± 4.46	10.00 ± 3.74	**11.25 ± 4.62 ***	**14.75 ± 2.77 ***	21.38 ± 5.71	**8.75 ± 4.85 ***	**10.31 ± 5.46 ***
MSH3 rs26279									
Thr/Thr	5.50 ± 3.63	8.90 ± 3.81	9.90 ± 7.09	10.13 ± 1.64	8.00 ± 2.73	16.88 ± 5.79	**19.00 ± 4.93**	6.61 ± 3.42	12.44 ± 6.18
Thr/Ala + Ala/Ala	4.80 ± 4.03	8.60 ± 6.54	7.00 ± 1.58	8.33 ± 5.13	14.00 ± 7.00	18.33 ± 3.51	**27.00 ± 2.00 ***	8.25 ± 6.78	12.25 ± 7.31
MSH4 rs5745325									
Ala/Ala	5.18 ± 3.79	8.91 ± 5.07	9.09 ± 6.64	9.63 ± 3.34	13.25 ± 5.68	13.75 ± 3.50	25.50 ± 4.73	7.33 ± 5.55	10.20 ± 5.09
Ala/Thr + Thr/Thr	5.50 ± 3.70	8.50 ± 3.87	8.50 ± 4.04	9.67 ± 0.58	7.57 ± 2.88	19.29 ± 4.99	18.67 ± 4.68	6.82 ± 3.19	**15.36 ± 7.00 ***
NBN rs1805794									
Glu/Glu	5.43 ± 4.61	10.00 ± 4.51	8.14 ± 4.56	9.86 ± 2.12	9.00 ± 4.84	**19.13 ± 4.64**	19.57 ± 4.89	7.33 ± 4.92	14.87 ± 6.46
Glu/Gln + Gln/Gln	5.13 ± 2.85	7.75 ± 4.80	9.63 ± 7.15	9.25 ± 4.11	11.33 ± 5.13	**12.33 ± 2.52 ***	25.67 ± 5.77	6.82 ± 4.40	**9.00 ± 4.69 ***

* $p < 0.05$; p-value for variant allele carriers *versus* common allele homozygotes determined by the Student t test (whenever a normal distribution could not be excluded through the Shapiro-Wilk test) or the Mann-Whitney U test (remaining cases). Significant findings highlighted in bold.

Table 5. Variation in the frequency of micronucleated cells from baseline (‰BNMN, mean ± SD) in each ^{131}I dose group at t_1, t_3/t_6, and t_{24}, according to genotype (only SNPs presenting significant findings are shown).

Genotype	70 mCi Group (n = 15), ‰BNMN (mean ± SD)			100 mCi Group (n = 11), ‰BNMN (mean ± SD)		70 + 100 mCi Groups (n = 26), ‰BNMN (mean ± SD)
	Δt_1	Δt_6	Δt_{24}	Δt_1	Δt_3	Δt_1
MLH1 rs1799977						
Ile/Ile	8.00 ± 4.97	6.71 ± 6.85	5.00 ± 3.39	18.67 ± 3.06	16.50 ± 6.36	11.20 ± 6.71
Ile/Val + Val/Val	−0.38 ± 3.70 *	1.00 ± 4.90	3.50 ± 4.37	3.50 ± 4.57 *	10.13 ± 5.28	1.56 ± 4.49 *
MSH4 rs5745325						
Ala/Ala	3.73 ± 6.83	3.91 ± 7.05	4.13 ± 3.91	0.50 ± 3.11	12.25 ± 5.32	2.87 ± 6.13
Ala/Thr + Thr/Thr	3.00 ± 3.56	3.00 ± 4.90	4.33 ± 4.51	11.71 ± 7.27 *	10.83 ± 6.49	8.55 ± 7.41 *

* $p < 0.05$; p-value for variant allele carriers *versus* common allele homozygotes determined by the Student t test (whenever a normal distribution could not be excluded through the Shapiro-Wilk test) or the Mann-Whitney U test (remaining cases). Significant findings highlighted in bold.

One month after ^{131}I administration, *MLH1* rs1799977 variant allele carriers always presented significantly lower BNMN levels than patients homozygous for the common allele, either when considering absolute values ($p = 0.004$, $p = 0.012$ and $p = 0.034$ in the 70 mCi, 100 mCi, and in the pool of both groups, respectively) or the net variation from baseline ($p = 0.002$, $p = 0.001$ and $p < 0.001$ in the 70 mCi, 100 mCi and in the pool of both groups, respectively). BNMN frequency one month after therapy was also significantly lower in carriers of the variant allele for *NBN* rs1805794 ($p = 0.043$ in the 100 mCi group and $p = 0.017$ in the pool of both groups), with the difference in net BNMN values almost being significant ($p = 0.099$ in the 100 mCi dose group and $p = 0.058$ in the pool of both groups). Further, carriers of at least one *MSH4* rs5745325 variant allele exhibited higher levels of ^{131}I-induced BNMN than patients homozygous for the common allele ($p = 0.018$ in the 100 mCi group, $p = 0.043$ in the combination of both groups), with the difference in absolute BNMN frequencies being significant in the pooled analysis of both groups ($p = 0.039$) and almost significant in the 100 mCi group ($p = 0.084$).

Three months after therapy, significantly higher BNMN frequencies were found in patients from the 100 mCi group carrying the *MSH3* rs26279 variant allele ($p = 0.030$).

No other significant difference in either absolute or therapy-induced BNMN frequencies was found between the different genotypes of the DNA repair SNPs, at any time point. Likewise, no influence of genotype in CBPI, either absolute or relative to baseline values, was detected for any of the DNA repair SNPs considered in this study, at any time point (Table S6).

4. Discussion

We have previously demonstrated a significant increase in BNMN frequency in peripheral lymphocytes from 19 DTC patients treated with 70 mCi ^{131}I [22]. In the present exploratory study, in order to confirm these findings, to evaluate the long-term persistence of such ^{131}I-induced DNA damage and to determine whether it may be influenced by DNA repair SNPs, we extended our analysis at 2 years after ^{131}I administration in this group of patients, included a new group of patients submitted to RAI therapy with 100 mCi and profiled 9 DNA repair SNPs in patients from both groups.

In line with our previously reported results, we observed, in the 100 mCi dose group, a significant and persistent increase in BNMN frequency after ^{131}I therapy, with mean levels being always higher than in the 70 mCi group, irrespective of the time point considered. Replication across two independent sets of patients and observation of a dose effect strongly suggests a causal relation between RAI therapy and systemic chromosomal damage in lymphocytes, as assessed by the MNCB assay. Such correlation has been repeatedly demonstrated (both in thyroid patients following RAI therapy [27–32] and in other settings where exposure to low levels of low-LET (linear energy transfer) ionizing radiation occurs [28,33]) and is expected since ^{131}I may be taken up by extra-thyroidal cells [7] and emit β- and γ-radiation capable of inducing dose-dependent chromosomal damage detectable by cytogenetic analysis (e.g., micronuclei) [27,28,32]. The ability of ^{131}I to induce cytogenetic damage in peripheral lymphocytes in a dose-dependent manner is, in fact, clear and well-established, allowing BNMN frequency to be used as a valid, highly sensitive, and specific biomarker of effect for biological dosimetry of RAI therapy and, hence, to predict its associated genotoxic risk in dividing mammalian cells [27,28,32,34,35].

A less clear picture exists, however, concerning the long-term persistence (kinetics of the recovery) of such IR-induced cytogenetic damage. Our results from the 70 mCi dose group suggest that ^{131}I-induced damage in peripheral lymphocytes persists for at least 2 years. Despite negative results have also been published [36,37], our results are in line with most prior follow-up studies on RAI therapy or other low-dose IR exposures (e.g., for diagnostic purposes) [28,29,38–41]. Considering the half-life of ^{131}I (ranging from 1 to 8 days in thyroidectomized and non-thyroidectomized TC patients, respectively) [28] and of circulating lymphocytes (about 3 years) [28,38], such repeated demonstration of persistent cytogenetic damage is somehow surprising and challenge the widely held views about the mechanisms of IR-induced DNA damage. Possible explanations for the long-term genomic instability of lymphocytes from ^{131}I-exposed subjects include the introduction, upon irradiation, of DNA damage and cytogenetic alterations (1) in a subset of long-lived naïve T lymphocytes, quiescent cells that survive for prolonged periods of time in a resting stage, retaining the initially inflicted DNA damage and expressing it as micronuclei when stimulated to proliferate in the CBMN assay [38,42,43], (2) in hematopoietic stem and progenitor cells that, through clonal expansion, may give rise to mature T lymphocytes with stable and unstable aberrations, perpetuating genomic instability in time (transgenerational effect) [38,42,43], and (3) in non-irradiated lymphocytes (a delayed non-targeted effect), as a result of the long-term production and plasma secretion of soluble clastogenic factors by irradiated cells (oxidative stress by-products such as ROS (reactive oxygen species) and inflammatory cytokines such as TNF-α) that may further extend IR-induced cytogenetic damage in time ("bystander effect") [44]. The two latter explanations are generally favored, as a large number of studies exist demonstrating either the high frequency of gene mutations and chromosomal aberrations in the progeny of irradiated cells or the production and plasma release of factors with clastogenic activity by irradiated cells (including one on ^{131}I-treated patients) [37]. Overall, current evidence [44–47] supports the notion that a potent long-term inflammatory-type response develops upon IR exposure, irradiated cells producing danger signals (oxidative stress by-products and inflammatory cytokines) capable of exerting an array of persistent bystander effects in non-irradiated cells (altered levels of damage-inducible and stress-related proteins), leading to delayed genomic instability (chromosomal aberrations, sister chromatid exchanges, micronuclei formation/induction or mutations), hence, predisposing to malignancy (altered proliferation or transformation). Such long-term inflammatory-type response could also be responsible for the marked reduction in CBPI that we observed at 24 months after ^{131}I therapy.

In this study, complying with current recommendations, we also investigated the role of potential confounding factors on BNMN frequency. As reviewed elsewhere [48–50] and demonstrated through meta-analysis in the International Human MicroNucleus (HUMN) Project [51], age and gender are well-established factors, with increasing age and female gender being consistently associated with higher BNMN levels in peripheral blood lymphocytes. The influence of age has been demonstrated, in particular, in ^{131}I-treated patients [28,31]. Data on the potential role of smoking status on BNMN levels are somewhat more inconsistent, and many studies failing to find an association except, maybe, in heavy smokers and in those with relevant occupational exposures [48–51]. In this study, no significant effect of gender, age, or smoking habits on BNMN levels or its net balance was detected, irrespective of the time point or dose group. The study was probably underpowered to detect such effects. It is also possible that the effect of these variables may have been masked by the impact of internal IR exposure after ^{131}I administration.

We did observe, however, in the 70 mCi group only, differences on BNMN levels between the two TC histotypes, as FTC patients presented significantly higher basal BNMN frequency than PTC patients but significantly lower therapy-induced BNMN levels at one month after ^{131}I administration. This is suggestive of higher background genomic instability in FTC but higher sensitivity to the DNA damaging effects of IR in PTC. Considering the small sample size and the non-reproducibility of the findings between the two dose groups, extreme caution must be taken in the interpretation of these results. Nevertheless, the available evidence supports both findings: PTC usually presents as a microsatellite stable tumor, with no appreciable levels of either loss of heterozygosity (LOH) or aneuploidy (stable chromosome profile) [52–54]. On the contrary, a considerable degree of chromosomal instability appears to be a hallmark feature of FTC, which presents a consistently higher frequency of chromosomal abnormalities, LOH, allelic loss, and a higher mutational burden compared to PTC [52,53,55–57]. Microsatellite instability (MSI), despite uncommon in TC, also appears to be more frequent in FTC than in PTC [53–55]. The available evidence thus largely supports our observation of higher background genomic instability in FTC. Moreover, considering that activating *RAS* mutations are commonly observed in FTC but not in PTC [53,58,59], the association between increased *RAS* expression and decreased frequency of IR-induced MN reported by Miller et al. [60] is coherent with our own observation of lower ^{131}I-induced BNMN frequency in FTC, supporting the idea that this histotype is less sensitive to the DNA damaging effects of IR than PTC. Such hypothesis (i.e., higher sensitivity to

IR in PTC) is further reinforced by a recent observation, through meta-analysis, of increased efficacy of RAI therapy in PTC patients, compared to FTC [61] but more studies are needed for a solid conclusion to be drawn.

Moreover, in the present study, we further evaluated the potential impact of selected HR, NHEJ, and MMR pathway SNPs on BNMN levels, before and after the administration of ^{131}I. To our knowledge, this is the first study doing so. Significant genotype effects on MN frequency and/or its net balance were observed for HR (*NBN*) and MMR (*MLH1*, *MSH3*, *MSH4*) repair pathway SNPs across different time points. This was expected because (1) IR exposure results in increased DNA damage, most notably, single- and double-strand breaks, oxidative lesions (e.g., 8-oxoG), DNA-protein crosslinks (DPCs) and clustered DNA lesions [62–67]; (2) the HR pathway, acting in the S/G2 stages of the cell cycle, is the major DNA repair pathway involved in the error-free correction of DSBs [11,33,35,68]; (3) MMR proteins, besides their canonical actions on the post-replication repair of mispaired nucleotides and insertion–deletion loops, have also been demonstrated to play an important role on the damage response to IR-induced DSBs, either through cooperation with HR or through signaling for cell-cycle arrest and apoptosis [64,69–71]; (4) DSBs, if left unrepaired, e.g., due to the presence of SNPs that reduce the DNA repair capacity, may give rise to chromosome breakage and MN formation upon replication [28,33,35,72]. The potential influence of functional DSB repair SNPs on ^{131}I-induced BNMN frequency is, therefore, fully justified. A literature review on the functional impact of these SNPs and their putative association with response to radio and/or chemotherapy was performed and is presented below (Table 6).

Table 6. Literature review on the functional impact of the studied SNPs and their putative association with radio and/or chemosensitivity (only SNPs presenting significant findings in the present study are shown).

Gene	DB SNP Cluster ID (RS NO.)	Functional Impact	Clinical Association Studies (Radio and/or Chemosensitivity)
MLH1	rs1799977	Missense SNP located in a highly conserved N-terminal ATPase domain, vital for MLH1 function [73]; G allele associated with reduced expression [74–77].	GG genotype associated with increased radiosensitivity in cancer patients, translating into increased efficacy [78] or toxicity [79] of radiotherapy (alone or combined with chemotherapy).
MSH3	rs26279	Missense SNP located in the ATPase domain, critical for protein activity [80]; altered expression has been suggested [81] but not confirmed [82].	GG genotype associated with decreased incidence of radiation dermatitis in breast cancer patients receiving radiotherapy [83], decreased overall survival in head and neck squamous cell carcinoma patients submitted to radiochemotherapy [81] and decreased response to platinum-based chemotherapy in advanced non-small cell lung cancer patients [84].
MSH4	rs5745325	Missense SNP located in the N-terminal domain, involved in the interaction with eIF3f [85].	None to be reported.
NBN	rs1805794	Missense SNP located in the BRCT domain, a region involved in the interaction with BRCA1 [86–89]; conflicting results from functional studies [88,90–92].	No association detected in most studies focusing on response to radiotherapy [79,93–96] or chemotherapy [97–99]; conflicting results also reported as the C allele has been associated with either improved [86,100] or worse [68,101] prognosis upon platinum-based chemotherapy; increased frequency of binucleated lymphocytes with nucleoplasmic bridges in Glu/Gln children with high IR exposure, opposite to Gln/Gln children [102].

MLH1, together with PMS2, forms the MutLα heterodimer, a complex critical for the maintenance of genomic integrity [103,104]. The common rs1799977 (c.665A>G, Ile219Val) missense SNP is located in a region that codes for a highly conserved N-terminal ATPase domain, vital for MLH1 function. However, since both alleles code for nonpolar pH-neutral amino acids, the substitution is considered conservative and not expected to result in drastic changes in protein properties and function [73].

Several functional studies support this hypothesis [73,74,105–107] but the existence of a more subtle effect should not be excluded [73,106,108,109] as an association between the G variant allele and reduced MLH1 expression has been demonstrated repeatedly in cancer patients [74–77]. Moreover, two recent meta-analyses have associated this variant with increased risk of colorectal cancer [110,111]. Considering the important role that MLH1 plays in the maintenance of genome integrity and cancer avoidance, both observations are compatible with our own observation of increased baseline BNMN levels in TC patients carrying the G allele. A different picture emerges, however, upon IR exposure: as previously stated, MMR proteins such as MLH1 play a dual role in the DNA damage response to IR, triggering cell-cycle arrest and allowing for either DSB repair or apoptosis [11,64]. MMR proficiency is thus expected to result in higher repair efficiency of IR-induced damage (hence, lower cytogenetic levels) and, simultaneously, higher cytotoxicity upon IR exposure (hence, increased sensitivity to radiotherapy). Indeed, alongside with increased cancer susceptibility, the *MLH1* rs1799977 variant GG genotype has been associated with increased radiosensitivity in cancer patients, translating into increased efficacy [78] or toxicity [79] of radiotherapy (alone or combined with chemotherapy). This is suggestive of increased MMR proficiency in such patients and supports our own observation of significantly lower BNMN levels, one month after ^{131}I therapy, in TC patients carrying the G allele. How the same allele may be associated with decreased function under basal conditions and increased function after IR exposure remains to be explained: MLH1 has been demonstrated to be upregulated upon IR exposure [112,113], it is possible that such upregulation might be more pronounced in G allele carriers, but this is highly speculative. Nevertheless, the high level of significance in our observations (especially when considering the change in MN frequency from baseline) and their cross-validation in independent groups strengthen our conclusions and warrant further studies to clarify this issue.

Two other MMR polymorphisms presented significant findings in our study, *MSH3* rs26279 and *MSH4* rs5745325. Like MLH1, MSH3 also appears to be involved in the repair and damage response to IR-associated lesions such as DSBs and inter-strand crosslinks [84,114]. *MSH3* rs26279 (c.3133A>G; Thr1045Ala) is a common SNP that results in an amino acid change in the ATPase domain of MLH3. This domain is critical for MSH3 activity, suggesting a functional impact for this variant [80]. Such hypothesis remains to be verified as, to the best of our knowledge, functional studies are lacking. An association with altered MSH3 expression levels has been suggested [81] but not confirmed [82]. The *MSH3* rs26279 G allele or GG genotype has been consistently associated with cancer risk in all 3 meta-analysis that we are aware of, particularly for colon and breast cancer [115–117], suggesting decreased DNA repair capacity in G allele carriers. Further, *MSH3* rs26279 GG homozygosity has also been associated with decreased incidence of radiation dermatitis in breast cancer patients receiving radiotherapy [83], decreased overall survival in head and neck squamous cell carcinoma patients submitted to radiochemotherapy [81], and decreased response to platinum-based chemotherapy in advanced non-small cell lung cancer patients [84], suggesting decreased sensitivity to DNA damaging agents such as IR or platinum in GG homozygous individuals. Such phenotype is commonly associated with MMR deficiency [64,69,70,118,119]. If we consider, once again, the dual role that MMR proteins such as MSH3 play in damage repair and apoptosis, these results are compatible with decreased G allele function, resulting in decreased DNA repair and apoptosis, increased damage tolerance, resistance to radio/chemotherapy, and reduced efficacy and cytotoxicity of such therapeutic agents. Our own observation of increased MN levels in TC patients carrying the G allele, 6 months after receiving 100 mCi ^{131}I, fits comfortably into this picture.

Likewise, in our study, MN frequency was also significantly increased (absolute and change from baseline values) in TC patients carrying the A allele of *MSH4* rs5745325, one month after ^{131}I administration. *MSH4* rs5745325 (c.289G>A; Ala97Thr) has only seldom been evaluated: on single SNP analysis, two prior studies by our team failed to detect an association with either thyroid [21] or breast cancer risk [120]. The same was observed in the only two other association studies that we found focusing on this SNP [121,122]. Interestingly, in three out of these four studies, significant associations were detected when interactions with other SNPs—*MSH6* rs1042821 [21], *MLH3* rs175080 [120], and *CHRNA5* rs16969968 [121]—were considered. Besides the important role that MSH4 plays in recombinational repair during meiosis [123], it is also suggested to participate, through interaction with a vast array of binding partners, in DSB-triggered damage response and repair [85,123,124]. It is possible that *MSH4* rs5745325 interferes with the binding properties of MSH4, with impact on its putative contribution to the DNA damage response and repair. The interaction of MSH4 with eIF3f (a subunit of the eIF3 complex implicated in apoptosis regulation and tumor development), for example, occurs at the region comprising the first 150 amino acids of the N-terminal domain of MSH4 (where rs5745325 is located) and has been demonstrated to foster hMSH4 stabilization and to modulate sensitivity to IR-induced DNA damage [85]. This is in line with our own findings.

Finally, we also observed a significant association between *NBN* rs1805794 and BNMN frequency, one month after the administration of 100 mCi ^{131}I. Nibrin plays a pivotal role in the initial steps of the cellular response to DNA damage, directly initiating DSB repair through the RAD51-dependent HR pathway and further contributing to cell cycle checkpoint activation through an ATM-dependent pathway [68,125–127]. Inactivating germline mutations in the *NBN* gene (which encodes for the Nibrin protein) markedly impair DSB repair and cause the Nijmegen breakage syndrome, characterized by chromosomal instability, increased cancer susceptibility, and increased sensitivity to DSB-causing agents such as IR or cisplatin. These features highlight the importance of Nibrin for genome stability (hence, cancer prevention) [86,93,125,127]. NBN overexpression also appears to be associated with poor prognosis in several types of cancer [68], which is consistent with a putative increase in DNA repair efficiency, hence, resistance to cytotoxic therapy. Among the numerous *NBN* polymorphisms, rs1805794 (c.553G>C; Glu185Gln) is the most frequently investigated. This missense variant results in an amino acid change in the BRCT (BRCA1 C Terminus) domain (amino acids 108-196), a domain involved in the interaction of Nibrin with BRCA1. The resulting complex (the BRCA1-associated genome surveillance complex, BASC) is responsible for the recognition and repair of aberrant DNA [86–89]. *NBN* rs1805794 has been suggested to interfere with the interaction properties of Nibrin and thus with DNA repair capacity, sensitivity to DNA damaging agents (such as IR) and cancer susceptibility. Accordingly, *NBN* rs1805794 has been repeatedly associated with cancer risk, as demonstrated by numerous meta-analysis [68,88,89,125,128–132] but conflicting reports exist [126,127,133,134]. Interestingly, the association may vary according to ethnicity [88,130] and tumor site [125], as one of these meta-analysis has demonstrated, for example, increased risk of leukemia, nasopharyngeal, and urinary system cancers but decreased risk of lung, gastric, and digestive system cancers [125]. Furthermore, final conclusive evidence on the significance of *NBN* rs1805794 is still lacking, as the functional studies performed thus far have yielded negative or conflicting results: while lymphocytes from healthy individuals homozygous for the G allele have been reported to present higher DNA damage levels (as assessed by the Comet assay) than lymphocytes from C allele carriers [90], opposite results have been reported in ex vivo X-ray irradiated cells from healthy subjects [88]. Further ex vivo irradiation studies have failed to observe a significant influence of *NBN* rs1805794 on DNA repair capacity and radiosensitivity [91,92]. Furthermore, since a putative functional impact of this SNP on DNA repair capacity could possibly influence patient sensitivity to radio and/or chemotherapy, association studies correlating *NBN* rs1805794 genotype with therapy response, toxicity, or prognosis have also been performed. Again, most studies failed to find an association in radiotherapy [79,93–96] or chemotherapy [97–99] treated patients, while other studies presented opposite findings, associating the *NBN* rs1805794 C allele with either improved [86,100] or worse [68,101] prognosis upon platinum-based chemotherapy. Interestingly, increased frequency of binucleated lymphocytes with nucleoplasmic bridges was observed in peripheral lymphocytes from children with high environmental exposure to IR that were heterozygous for *NBN* rs1805794, while the reverse patter was observed in children homozygous for the Gln allele [102]. This may be suggestive of molecular heterosis, a hypothesis that, considering the high interethnic variability of the *NBN* rs1805794 distribution, could help in explaining such divergent results. Overall, despite extensively investigated, the functional significance of *NBN* rs1805794, as well as its putative role in

5. Conclusions

In conclusion, our results confirm that BNMN levels in peripheral lymphocytes from DTC patients increase significantly immediately 1 month after ^{131}I therapy and further suggest that these remain stable and persistently higher than baseline for at least 2 years. Furthermore, a marked reduction in CBPI is observed at 24 months after ^{131}I administration. Moreover, HR and MMR SNPs (*MLH1* rs1799977, *MSH3* rs26279, *MSH4* rs5745325, and *NBN* rs1805794) were, for the first time, associated with IR-induced MN, a cytogenetic marker of DNA damage, in TC patients submitted to ^{131}I therapy. Among such findings, a highly significant and independently replicated association was observed for *MLH1* rs1799977, strongly suggesting a role for this particular SNP on the personalization of RAI therapy in TC cancer patients. Baseline and post-therapy MN levels also diverged according to tumor histotype. These results should be regarded as merely suggestive and proof of concept, as the sample was small and the number of tests was high, increasing the likelihood of false-positive results. Nevertheless, our findings suggest that TC therapy with ^{131}I may pose a long-term challenge to cells other than thyrocytes and that the patient genetic profile may influence the individual sensitivity to this therapy. Such hypotheses are of relevance to the efficacy and safety of ^{131}I therapy, a widespread practice in TC patients. As such, extending the benefit already achieved with the latest guidelines on TC treatment in terms of risk/benefit ratio through improved clinical assessment of the potential long-term risks of ^{131}I therapy is desirable. Likewise, despite the micronucleus test is considered the gold standard methodology in genetic toxicology testing and often used as a "stand-alone" test in numerous and relevant papers in this area, other tests should also be employed to validate these results. Furthermore, potential radiogenomic markers such as those suggested here should be evaluated in larger samples, preferentially through multi-center independent studies adequately powered to provide more robust evidence and, eventually, to allow for gene-gene and gene-environment interactions to be assessed. Identifying the most clinically relevant variables, genetic or non-genetic, and accurately estimating their impact on ^{131}I therapy response rate and adverse event risk for each individual TC patient is the ultimate goal, under a personalized medicine approach.

Supplementary Materials: The following are available online at http://www.mdpi.com/2073-4425/11/9/1083/s1, Table S1: Allele and genotype frequencies in thyroid cancer patients submitted to ^{131}I therapy ($n = 26$) and in the original (reference) DTC population ($n = 106$), Table S2: BNMN frequency (‰, mean ± S.D.) in DTC patients before and after (1, 3/6, and 24 months) therapy with different doses of ^{131}I (70 and 100 mCi), Table S3: Frequency of micronucleated cells (‰ BNMN, mean ± SD) in the 70 mCi dose group at t_0, t_1, t_6 and t_{24}, and corresponding variation, according to genotype, Table S4: Frequency of micronucleated cells (‰ BNMN, mean ± SD) in the 100 mCi dose group at t_0, t_1 and t_3, and corresponding variation, according to genotype, Table S5: Frequency of micronucleated cells (‰ BNMN, mean ± SD) in the combined dose groups at t_0 and t_1, and corresponding variation, according to genotype, Table S6: Cytokinesis-Block Proliferation Index (CBPI, mean ± SD) in the 70 mCi dose group at t_0, t_1, t_6 and t_{24}, and corresponding variation, according to genotype.

Author Contributions: Conceptualization was mainly developed by J.R., T.C.F., and E.L.; methodology was performed by, O.M.G., L.S.S., and B.C.G.; validation proceedings by L.S.S., B.C.G., and S.N.S.; formal analysis was done by L.S.S. and S.N.S.; investigation was mainly performed by L.S.S. and B.C.G.; resources acquired in restrict collaboration by O.M.G. and T.C.F.; data curation, O.M.G., T.C.F., and E.L.; writing—original draft preparation, L.S.S.; writing—review and editing, B.C.G., O.M.G., S.N.S., and J.R.; visualization has been prepared by L.S.S. and S.N.S.; supervision of this project was done by J.R.; project administration, J.R. and E.L.; funding acquisition, J.R. All authors have read and agreed to the published version of the manuscript.

Funding: This research was funded by FCT—Fundação para a Ciência e a Tecnologia (Portuguese Foundation for Science and Technology) through Project UID/BIM/00009/2019—Centre for Toxicogenomics and Human Health.

Acknowledgments: The authors warmly acknowledge the generous collaboration of patients and controls in this study as well as of our colleague Ana Paula Azevedo for technical support.

Conflicts of Interest: The authors declare no conflict of interest. The funders had no role in the design of the study; in the collection, analyses, or interpretation of data; in the writing of the manuscript, or in the decision to publish the results.

References

1. Ferlay, J.; Ervik, M.; Lam, F.; Colombet, M.; Mery, L.; Piñeros, M.; Znaor, A.; Soerjomataram, I.; Bray, F. Global Cancer Observatory: Cancer Today. Available online: https://gco.iarc.fr/today (accessed on 28 May 2019).
2. Kitahara, C.M.; Sosa, J.A. The changing incidence of thyroid cancer. *Nat. Rev. Endocrinol.* **2016**, *12*, 646–653. [CrossRef] [PubMed]
3. Lebastchi, A.H.; Callender, G.G. Thyroid cancer. *Curr. Probl. Cancer* **2014**, *38*, 48–74. [CrossRef] [PubMed]
4. Khosravi, M.H.; Kouhi, A.; Saeedi, M.; Bagherihagh, A.; Amirzade-Iranaq, M.H. Thyroid Cancers: Considerations, Classifications, and Managements. In *Diagnosis and Management of Head and Neck Cancer*; Akarslan, Z., Ed.; IntechOpen: London, UK, 2017; pp. 57–82. [CrossRef]
5. Wild, C.; Weiderpass, E.; Stewart, B. (Eds.) *World Cancer Report: Cancer Research for Cancer Prevention*; International Agency for Research on Cancer: Lyon, France, 2020.
6. Mayson, S.E.; Yoo, D.C.; Gopalakrishnan, G. The evolving use of radioiodine therapy in differentiated thyroid cancer. *Oncology* **2015**, *88*, 247–256. [CrossRef]
7. Carballo, M.; Quiros, R.M. To treat or not to treat: The role of adjuvant radioiodine therapy in thyroid cancer patients. *J. Oncol.* **2012**, *2012*, 707156. [CrossRef] [PubMed]
8. Haugen, B.R.; Alexander, E.K.; Bible, K.C.; Doherty, G.M.; Mandel, S.J.; Nikiforov, Y.E.; Pacini, F.; Randolph, G.W.; Sawka, A.M.; Schlumberger, M.; et al. 2015 American Thyroid Association Management Guidelines for Adult Patients with Thyroid Nodules and Differentiated Thyroid Cancer: The American Thyroid Association Guidelines Task Force on Thyroid Nodules and Differentiated Thyroid Cancer. *Thyroid Off. J. Am. Thyroid Assoc.* **2016**, *26*, 1–133. [CrossRef] [PubMed]
9. Haugen, B.R. 2015 American Thyroid Association Management Guidelines for Adult Patients with Thyroid Nodules and Differentiated Thyroid Cancer: What is new and what has changed? *Cancer* **2017**, *123*, 372–381. [CrossRef]
10. Chatterjee, N.; Walker, G.C. Mechanisms of DNA damage, repair, and mutagenesis. *Environ. Mol. Mutagenesis* **2017**, *58*, 235–263. [CrossRef]
11. Collins, S.P.; Dritschilo, A. The mismatch repair and base excision repair pathways: An opportunity for individualized (personalized) sensitization of cancer therapy. *Cancer Biol. Ther.* **2009**, *8*, 1164–1166. [CrossRef]
12. Doai, M.; Watanabe, N.; Takahashi, T.; Taniguchi, M.; Tonami, H.; Iwabuchi, K.; Kayano, D.; Fukuoka, M.; Kinuya, S. Sensitive immunodetection of radiotoxicity after iodine-131 therapy for thyroid cancer using gamma-H2AX foci of DNA damage in lymphocytes. *Ann. Nucl. Med.* **2013**, *27*, 233–238. [CrossRef]
13. Eberlein, U.; Scherthan, H.; Bluemel, C.; Peper, M.; Lapa, C.; Buck, A.K.; Port, M.; Lassmann, M. DNA Damage in Peripheral Blood Lymphocytes of Thyroid Cancer Patients After Radioiodine Therapy. *J. Nucl. Med. Off. Publ. Soc. Nucl. Med.* **2016**, *57*, 173–179. [CrossRef]
14. Simonelli, V.; Mazzei, F.; D'Errico, M.; Dogliotti, E. Gene susceptibility to oxidative damage: From single nucleotide polymorphisms to function. *Mutat. Res.* **2012**, *731*, 1–13. [CrossRef] [PubMed]
15. Sameer, A.S.; Nissar, S. XPD-The Lynchpin of NER: Molecule, Gene, Polymorphisms, and Role in Colorectal Carcinogenesis. *Front. Mol. Biosci.* **2018**, *5*, 23. [CrossRef]
16. Adjadj, E.; Schlumberger, M.; de Vathaire, F. Germ-line DNA polymorphisms and susceptibility to differentiated thyroid cancer. *Lancet Oncol.* **2009**, *10*, 181–190. [CrossRef]
17. Gatzidou, E.; Michailidi, C.; Tseleni-Balafouta, S.; Theocharis, S. An epitome of DNA repair related genes and mechanisms in thyroid carcinoma. *Cancer Lett.* **2010**, *290*, 139–147. [CrossRef] [PubMed]
18. Santos, L.S.; Gomes, B.C.; Bastos, H.N.; Gil, O.M.; Azevedo, A.P.; Ferreira, T.C.; Limbert, E.; Silva, S.N.; Rueff, J. Thyroid Cancer: The Quest for Genetic Susceptibility Involving DNA Repair Genes. *Genes* **2019**, *10*, 586. [CrossRef]
19. Bastos, H.N.; Antao, M.R.; Silva, S.N.; Azevedo, A.P.; Manita, I.; Teixeira, V.; Pina, J.E.; Gil, O.M.; Ferreira, T.C.; Limbert, E.; et al. Association of polymorphisms in genes of the homologous recombination DNA repair pathway and thyroid cancer risk. *Thyroid Off. J. Am. Thyroid Assoc.* **2009**, *19*, 1067–1075. [CrossRef]
20. Gomes, B.C.; Silva, S.N.; Azevedo, A.P.; Manita, I.; Gil, O.M.; Ferreira, T.C.; Limbert, E.; Rueff, J.; Gaspar, J.F. The role of common variants of non-homologous end-joining repair genes XRCC4, LIG4 and Ku80 in thyroid cancer risk. *Oncol. Rep.* **2010**, *24*, 1079–1085.
21. Santos, L.S.; Silva, S.N.; Gil, O.M.; Ferreira, T.C.; Limbert, E.; Rueff, J. Mismatch repair single nucleotide polymorphisms and thyroid cancer susceptibility. *Oncol. Lett.* **2018**, *15*, 6715–6726. [CrossRef]

22. Gil, O.M.; Oliveira, N.G.; Rodrigues, A.S.; Laires, A.; Ferreira, T.C.; Limbert, E.; Leonard, A.; Gerber, G.; Rueff, J. Cytogenetic alterations and oxidative stress in thyroid cancer patients after iodine-131 therapy. *Mutagenesis* **2000**, *15*, 69–75. [CrossRef]
23. Monteiro Gil, O.; Oliveira, N.G.; Rodrigues, A.S.; Laires, A.; Ferreira, T.C.; Limbert, E.; Rueff, J. Possible transient adaptive response to mitomycin C in peripheral lymphocytes from thyroid cancer patients after iodine-131 therapy. *Int. J. Cancer* **2002**, *102*, 556–561. [CrossRef]
24. Gil, O.M.; Oliveira, N.G.; Rodrigues, A.S.; Laires, A.; Ferreira, T.C.; Limbert, E.; Rueff, J. No evidence of increased chromosomal aberrations and micronuclei in lymphocytes from nonfamilial thyroid cancer patients prior to radiotherapy. *Cancer Genet. Cytogenet.* **2000**, *123*, 55–60. [CrossRef] [PubMed]
25. Sole, X.; Guino, E.; Valls, J.; Iniesta, R.; Moreno, V. SNPStats: A web tool for the analysis of association studies. *Bioinformatics* **2006**, *22*, 1928–1929. [CrossRef] [PubMed]
26. OECD. *Test No. 487: In Vitro Mammalian Cell Micronucleus Test*; OECD: Paris, France, 2016. [CrossRef]
27. Hernández, A.; Xamena, N.; Gutiérrez, S.; Velázquez, A.; Creus, A.; Surrallés, J.; Galofré, P.; Marcos, R. Basal and induced micronucleus frequencies in human lymphocytes with different GST and NAT2 genetic backgrounds. *Mutat. Res.* **2006**, *606*, 12–20. [CrossRef]
28. Gutiérrez, S.; Carbonell, E.; Galofré, P.; Creus, A.; Marcos, R. Cytogenetic damage after 131-iodine treatment for hyperthyroidism and thyroid cancer. A study using the micronucleus test. *Eur. J. Nucl. Med.* **1999**, *26*, 1589–1596. [CrossRef] [PubMed]
29. Livingston, G.K.; Foster, A.E.; Elson, H.R. Effect of in vivo exposure to iodine-131 on the frequency and persistence of micronuclei in human lymphocytes. *J. Toxicol. Environ. Health* **1993**, *40*, 367–375. [CrossRef] [PubMed]
30. Ramírez, M.J.; Puerto, S.; Galofré, P.; Parry, E.M.; Parry, J.M.; Creus, A.; Marcos, R.; Surrallés, J. Multicolour FISH detection of radioactive iodine-induced 17cen-p53 chromosomal breakage in buccal cells from therapeutically exposed patients. *Carcinogenesis* **2000**, *21*, 1581–1586.
31. Ramírez, M.J.; Surrallés, J.; Galofré, P.; Creus, A.; Marcos, R. Radioactive iodine induces clastogenic and age-dependent aneugenic effects in lymphocytes of thyroid cancer patients as revealed by interphase FISH. *Mutagenesis* **1997**, *12*, 449–455. [CrossRef]
32. Monzen, S.; Mariya, Y.; Wojcik, A.; Kawamura, C.; Nakamura, A.; Chiba, M.; Hosoda, M.; Takai, Y. Predictive factors of cytotoxic damage in radioactive iodine treatment of differentiated thyroid cancer patients. *Mol. Clin. Oncol.* **2015**, *3*, 692–698. [CrossRef]
33. Shakeri, M.; Zakeri, F.; Changizi, V.; Rajabpour, M.R.; Farshidpour, M.R. Cytogenetic effects of radiation and genetic polymorphisms of the XRCC1 and XRCC3 repair genes in industrial radiographers. *Radiat. Environ. Biophys.* **2019**, *58*, 247–255. [CrossRef]
34. Müller, W.U.; Nüsse, M.; Miller, B.M.; Slavotinek, A.; Viaggi, S.; Streffer, C. Micronuclei: A biological indicator of radiation damage. *Mutat. Res.* **1996**, *366*, 163–169. [CrossRef]
35. Sinitsky, M.Y.; Minina, V.I.; Asanov, M.A.; Yuzhalin, A.E.; Ponasenko, A.V.; Druzhinin, V.G. Association of DNA repair gene polymorphisms with genotoxic stress in underground coal miners. *Mutagenesis* **2017**, *32*, 501–509. [CrossRef] [PubMed]
36. Watanabe, N.; Yokoyama, K.; Kinuya, S.; Shuke, N.; Shimizu, M.; Futatsuya, R.; Michigishi, T.; Tonami, N.; Seto, H.; Goodwin, D.A. Radiotoxicity after iodine-131 therapy for thyroid cancer using the micronucleus assay. *J. Nucl. Med. Off. Publ. Soc. Nucl. Med.* **1998**, *39*, 436–440.
37. Ballardin, M.; Gemignani, F.; Bodei, L.; Mariani, G.; Ferdeghini, M.; Rossi, A.M.; Migliore, L.; Barale, R. Formation of micronuclei and of clastogenic factor(s) in patients receiving therapeutic doses of iodine-131. *Mutat. Res.* **2002**, *514*, 77–85. [CrossRef]
38. Livingston, G.K.; Khvostunov, I.K. Cytogenetic effects of radioiodine therapy: A 20-year follow-up study. *Radiat. Environ. Biophys.* **2016**, *55*, 203–213. [CrossRef]
39. Puerto, S.; Marcos, R.; Ramírez, M.J.; Galofré, P.; Creus, A.; Surrallés, J. Equal induction and persistence of chromosome aberrations involving chromosomes 1, 4 and 10 in thyroid cancer patients treated with radioactive iodine. *Mutat. Res.* **2000**, *469*, 147–158. [CrossRef]
40. Fenech, M.; Denham, J.; Francis, W.; Morley, A. Micronuclei in cytokinesis-blocked lymphocytes of cancer patients following fractionated partial-body radiotherapy. *Int. J. Radiat. Biol.* **1990**, *57*, 373–383. [CrossRef]

41. M'Kacher, R.; Légal, J.D.; Schlumberger, M.; Aubert, B.; Beron-Gaillard, N.; Gaussen, A.; Parmentier, C. Sequential biological dosimetry after a single treatment with iodine-131 for differentiated thyroid carcinoma. *J. Nucl. Med. Off. Publ. Soc. Nucl. Med.* **1997**, *38*, 377–380.
42. Livingston, G.K.; Escalona, M.; Foster, A.; Balajee, A.S. Persistent in vivo cytogenetic effects of radioiodine therapy: A 21-year follow-up study using multicolor FISH. *J. Radiat. Res.* **2018**, *59*, 10–17. [CrossRef]
43. Livingston, G.K.; Ryan, T.L.; Smith, T.L.; Escalona, M.B.; Foster, A.E.; Balajee, A.S. Detection of Simple, Complex, and Clonal Chromosome Translocations Induced by Internal Radioiodine Exposure: A Cytogenetic Follow-Up Case Study after 25 Years. *Cytogenet. Genome Res.* **2019**, *159*, 169–181. [CrossRef]
44. Lindholm, C.; Acheva, A.; Salomaa, S. Clastogenic plasma factors: A short overview. *Radiat. Environ. Biophys.* **2010**, *49*, 133–138. [CrossRef]
45. Morgan, W.F. Is there a common mechanism underlying genomic instability, bystander effects and other nontargeted effects of exposure to ionizing radiation? *Oncogene* **2003**, *22*, 7094–7099. [CrossRef] [PubMed]
46. Mavragani, I.V.; Laskaratou, D.A.; Frey, B. Key mechanisms involved in ionizing radiation-induced systemic effects. A current review. *Toxicol. Res.* **2016**, *5*, 12–33. [CrossRef] [PubMed]
47. Lorimore, S.A.; McIlrath, J.M.; Coates, P.J.; Wright, E.G. Chromosomal instability in unirradiated hemopoietic cells resulting from a delayed in vivo bystander effect of gamma radiation. *Cancer Res.* **2005**, *65*, 5668–5673. [CrossRef] [PubMed]
48. Fenech, M.; Bonassi, S. The effect of age, gender, diet and lifestyle on DNA damage measured using micronucleus frequency in human peripheral blood lymphocytes. *Mutagenesis* **2011**, *26*, 43–49. [CrossRef]
49. Fenech, M.; Holland, N.; Zeiger, E.; Chang, W.P.; Burgaz, S.; Thomas, P.; Bolognesi, C.; Knasmueller, S.; Kirsch-Volders, M.; Bonassi, S. The HUMN and HUMNxL international collaboration projects on human micronucleus assays in lymphocytes and buccal cells–past, present and future. *Mutagenesis* **2011**, *26*, 239–245. [CrossRef]
50. Battershill, J.M.; Burnett, K.; Bull, S. Factors affecting the incidence of genotoxicity biomarkers in peripheral blood lymphocytes: Impact on design of biomonitoring studies. *Mutagenesis* **2008**, *23*, 423–437. [CrossRef]
51. Bonassi, S.; Fenech, M.; Lando, C.; Lin, Y.P.; Ceppi, M.; Chang, W.P.; Holland, N.; Kirsch-Volders, M.; Zeiger, E.; Ban, S.; et al. HUman MicroNucleus project: International database comparison for results with the cytokinesis-block micronucleus assay in human lymphocytes: I. Effect of laboratory protocol, scoring criteria, and host factors on the frequency of micronuclei. *Environ. Mol. Mutagenesis* **2001**, *37*, 31–45. [CrossRef]
52. Caria, P.; Vanni, R. Cytogenetic and molecular events in adenoma and well-differentiated thyroid follicular-cell neoplasia. *Cancer Genet. Cytogenet.* **2010**, *203*, 21–29. [CrossRef]
53. Genutis, L.K.; Tomsic, J.; Bundschuh, R.A.; Brock, P.L.; Williams, M.D.; Roychowdhury, S.; Reeser, J.W.; Frankel, W.L.; Alsomali, M.; Routbort, M.J.; et al. Microsatellite Instability Occurs in a Subset of Follicular Thyroid Cancers. *Thyroid Off. J. Am. Thyroid Assoc.* **2019**, *29*, 523–529. [CrossRef]
54. Lazzereschi, D.; Palmirotta, R.; Ranieri, A.; Ottini, L.; Veri, M.C.; Cama, A.; Cetta, F.; Nardi, F.; Colletta, G.; Mariani-Costantini, R. Microsatellite instability in thyroid tumours and tumour-like lesions. *Br. J. Cancer* **1999**, *79*, 340–345. [CrossRef]
55. Migdalska-Sek, M.; Czarnecka, K.H.; Kusinski, M.; Pastuszak-Lewandoska, D.; Nawrot, E.; Kuzdak, K.; Brzezianska-Lasota, E. Clinicopathological Significance of Overall Frequency of Allelic Loss (OFAL) in Lesions Derived from Thyroid Follicular Cell. *Mol. Diagn. Ther.* **2019**, *23*, 369–382. [CrossRef] [PubMed]
56. Ward, L.S.; Brenta, G.; Medvedovic, M.; Fagin, J.A. Studies of allelic loss in thyroid tumors reveal major differences in chromosomal instability between papillary and follicular carcinomas. *J. Clin. Endocrinol. Metab.* **1998**, *83*, 525–530. [CrossRef] [PubMed]
57. Gillespie, J.W.; Nasir, A.; Kaiser, H.E. Loss of heterozygosity in papillary and follicular thyroid carcinoma: A mini review. *VIVO (AthensGreece)* **2000**, *14*, 139–140.
58. Xing, M. Molecular pathogenesis and mechanisms of thyroid cancer. *Nat. Rev. Cancer* **2013**, *13*, 184–199. [CrossRef] [PubMed]
59. Sobrinho-Simoes, M.; Eloy, C.; Magalhaes, J.; Lobo, C.; Amaro, T. Follicular thyroid carcinoma. *Mod. Pathol.* **2011**, *24*, S10–S18. [CrossRef]
60. Miller, A.C.; Gafner, J.; Clark, E.P.; Samid, D. Differences in radiation-induced micronuclei yields of human cells: Influence of ras gene expression and protein localization. *Int. J. Radiat. Biol.* **1993**, *64*, 547–554. [CrossRef]

61. Zhang, X.; Liu, D.S.; Luan, Z.S.; Zhang, F.; Liu, X.H.; Zhou, W.; Zhong, S.F.; Lai, H. Efficacy of radioiodine therapy for treating 20 patients with pulmonary metastases from differentiated thyroid cancer and a meta-analysis of the current literature. *Clin. Transl. Oncol.* **2018**, *20*, 928–935. [CrossRef]

62. Eccles, L.J.; O'Neill, P.; Lomax, M.E. Delayed repair of radiation induced clustered DNA damage: Friend or foe? *Mutat. Res.* **2011**, *711*, 134–141. [CrossRef] [PubMed]

63. Sage, E.; Shikazono, N. Radiation-induced clustered DNA lesions: Repair and mutagenesis. *Free Radic. Biol. Med.* **2017**, *107*, 125–135. [CrossRef]

64. Martin, L.M.; Marples, B.; Coffey, M.; Lawler, M.; Lynch, T.H.; Hollywood, D.; Marignol, L. DNA mismatch repair and the DNA damage response to ionizing radiation: Making sense of apparently conflicting data. *Cancer Treat. Rev.* **2010**, *36*, 518–527. [CrossRef]

65. Nickoloff, J.A.; Sharma, N.; Taylor, L. Clustered DNA Double-Strand Breaks: Biological Effects and Relevance to Cancer Radiotherapy. *Genes* **2020**, *11*, 99. [CrossRef] [PubMed]

66. Zhang, H.; Xiong, Y.; Chen, J. DNA-protein cross-link repair: What do we know now? *Cell Biosci.* **2020**, *10*, 3. [CrossRef] [PubMed]

67. Nakano, T.; Xu, X.; Salem, A.M.H.; Shoulkamy, M.I.; Ide, H. Radiation-induced DNA-protein cross-links: Mechanisms and biological significance. *Free Radic. Biol. Med.* **2017**, *107*, 136–145. [CrossRef] [PubMed]

68. Wang, L.; Cheng, J.; Gao, J.; Wang, J.; Liu, X.; Xiong, L. Association between the NBS1 Glu185Gln polymorphism and lung cancer risk: A systemic review and meta-analysis. *Mol. Biol. Rep.* **2013**, *40*, 2711–2715. [CrossRef]

69. Kinsella, T.J. Coordination of DNA mismatch repair and base excision repair processing of chemotherapy and radiation damage for targeting resistant cancers. *Clin. Cancer Res. Off. J. Am. Assoc. Cancer Res.* **2009**, *15*, 1853–1859. [CrossRef]

70. Edelbrock, M.A.; Kaliyaperumal, S.; Williams, K.J. Structural, molecular and cellular functions of MSH2 and MSH6 during DNA mismatch repair, damage signaling and other noncanonical activities. *Mutat. Res.* **2013**, *743*, 53–66. [CrossRef]

71. Iyama, T.; Wilson, D.M., 3rd. DNA repair mechanisms in dividing and non-dividing cells. *DNA Repair* **2013**, *12*, 620–636. [CrossRef]

72. Iarmarcovai, G.; Bonassi, S.; Botta, A.; Baan, R.A.; Orsière, T. Genetic polymorphisms and micronucleus formation: A review of the literature. *Mutat. Res.* **2008**, *658*, 215–233. [CrossRef]

73. Plotz, G.; Raedle, J.; Spina, A.; Welsch, C.; Stallmach, A.; Zeuzem, S.; Schmidt, C. Evaluation of the MLH1 I219V alteration in DNA mismatch repair activity and ulcerative colitis. *Inflamm. Bowel Dis.* **2008**, *14*, 605–611. [CrossRef]

74. Milanizadeh, S.; Khanyaghma, M.; Haghighi, M.M.; Mohebbi, S.; Damavand, B.; Almasi, S.; Azimzadeh, P.; Zali, M. Molecular analysis of imperative polymorphisms of MLH1 gene in sporadic colorectal cancer. *Cancer Biomark. Sect. A Dis. Markers* **2013**, *13*, 427–432. [CrossRef]

75. Kim, J.C.; Roh, S.A.; Koo, K.H.; Ka, I.H.; Kim, H.C.; Yu, C.S.; Lee, K.H.; Kim, J.S.; Lee, H.I.; Bodmer, W.F. Genotyping possible polymorphic variants of human mismatch repair genes in healthy Korean individuals and sporadic colorectal cancer patients. *Fam. Cancer* **2004**, *3*, 129–137. [CrossRef] [PubMed]

76. Rossi, D.; Rasi, S.; Di Rocco, A.; Fabbri, A.; Forconi, F.; Gloghini, A.; Bruscaggin, A.; Franceschetti, S.; Fangazio, M.; De Paoli, L.; et al. The host genetic background of DNA repair mechanisms is an independent predictor of survival in diffuse large B-cell lymphoma. *Blood* **2011**, *117*, 2405–2413. [CrossRef] [PubMed]

77. Xiao, X.Q.; Gong, W.D.; Wang, S.Z.; Zhang, Z.D.; Rui, X.P.; Wu, G.Z.; Ren, F. Polymorphisms of mismatch repair gene hMLH1 and hMSH2 and risk of gastric cancer in a Chinese population. *Oncol. Lett.* **2012**, *3*, 591–598. [CrossRef] [PubMed]

78. Dreussi, E.; Cecchin, E.; Polesel, J.; Canzonieri, V.; Agostini, M.; Boso, C.; Belluco, C.; Buonadonna, A.; Lonardi, S.; Bergamo, F.; et al. Pharmacogenetics Biomarkers and Their Specific Role in Neoadjuvant Chemoradiotherapy Treatments: An Exploratory Study on Rectal Cancer Patients. *Int. J. Mol. Sci.* **2016**, *17*, 1482. [CrossRef]

79. Damaraju, S.; Murray, D.; Dufour, J.; Carandang, D.; Myrehaug, S.; Fallone, G.; Field, C.; Greiner, R.; Hanson, J.; Cass, C.E.; et al. Association of DNA repair and steroid metabolism gene polymorphisms with clinical late toxicity in patients treated with conformal radiotherapy for prostate cancer. *Clin. Cancer Res. Off. J. Am. Assoc. Cancer Res.* **2006**, *12*, 2545–2554. [CrossRef]

80. Morales, F.; Vásquez, M.; Santamaría, C.; Cuenca, P.; Corrales, E.; Monckton, D.G. A polymorphism in the MSH3 mismatch repair gene is associated with the levels of somatic instability of the expanded CTG repeat in the blood DNA of myotonic dystrophy type 1 patients. *DNA Repair* **2016**, *40*, 57–66. [CrossRef]
81. Nogueira, G.A.; Lourenço, G.J.; Oliveira, C.B.; Marson, F.A.; Lopes-Aguiar, L.; Costa, E.F.; Lima, T.R.; Liutti, V.T.; Leal, F.; Santos, V.C.; et al. Association between genetic polymorphisms in DNA mismatch repair-related genes with risk and prognosis of head and neck squamous cell carcinoma. *Int. J. Cancer* **2015**, *137*, 810–818. [CrossRef]
82. Vogelsang, M.; Wang, Y.; Veber, N.; Mwapagha, L.M.; Parker, M.I. The cumulative effects of polymorphisms in the DNA mismatch repair genes and tobacco smoking in oesophageal cancer risk. *PLoS ONE* **2012**, *7*, e36962. [CrossRef]
83. Mangoni, M.; Bisanzi, S.; Carozzi, F.; Sani, C.; Biti, G.; Livi, L.; Barletta, E.; Costantini, A.S.; Gorini, G. Association between genetic polymorphisms in the XRCC1, XRCC3, XPD, GSTM1, GSTT1, MSH2, MLH1, MSH3, and MGMT genes and radiosensitivity in breast cancer patients. *Int. J. Radiat. Oncol. Biol. Phys.* **2011**, *81*, 52–58. [CrossRef]
84. Xu, X.L.; Yao, Y.L.; Xu, W.Z.; Feng, J.G.; Mao, W.M. Correlation of MSH3 polymorphisms with response and survival in advanced non-small cell lung cancer patients treated with first-line platinum-based chemotherapy. *Genet. Mol. Res. Gmr* **2015**, *14*, 3525–3533. [CrossRef]
85. Chu, Y.L.; Wu, X.; Xu, Y.; Her, C. MutS homologue hMSH4: Interaction with eIF3f and a role in NHEJ-mediated DSB repair. *Mol. Cancer* **2013**, *12*, 51. [CrossRef] [PubMed]
86. Xu, J.L.; Hu, L.M.; Huang, M.D.; Zhao, W.; Yin, Y.M.; Hu, Z.B.; Ma, H.X.; Shen, H.B.; Shu, Y.Q. Genetic variants of NBS1 predict clinical outcome of platinum-based chemotherapy in advanced non-small cell lung cancer in Chinese. *Asian Pac. J. Cancer Prev. Apjcp* **2012**, *13*, 851–856. [CrossRef] [PubMed]
87. Smith, T.R.; Liu-Mares, W.; Van Emburgh, B.O.; Levine, E.A.; Allen, G.O.; Hill, J.W.; Reis, I.M.; Kresty, L.A.; Pegram, M.D.; Miller, M.S.; et al. Genetic polymorphisms of multiple DNA repair pathways impact age at diagnosis and TP53 mutations in breast cancer. *Carcinogenesis* **2011**, *32*, 1354–1360. [CrossRef] [PubMed]
88. Fang, W.; Qiu, F.; Zhang, L.; Deng, J.; Zhang, H.; Yang, L.; Zhou, Y.; Lu, J. The functional polymorphism of NBS1 p.Glu185Gln is associated with an increased risk of lung cancer in Chinese populations: Case-control and a meta-analysis. *Mutat. Res.* **2014**, *770*, 61–68. [CrossRef] [PubMed]
89. Lu, M.; Lu, J.; Yang, X.; Yang, M.; Tan, H.; Yun, B.; Shi, L. Association between the NBS1 E185Q polymorphism and cancer risk: A meta-analysis. *BMC Cancer* **2009**, *9*, 124. [CrossRef]
90. Goricar, K.; Erculj, N.; Zadel, M.; Dolzan, V. Genetic polymorphisms in homologous recombination repair genes in healthy Slovenian population and their influence on DNA damage. *Radiol. Oncol.* **2012**, *46*, 46–53. [CrossRef]
91. Gdowicz-Klosok, A.; Widel, M.; Rzeszowska-Wolny, J. The influence of XPD, APE1, XRCC1, and NBS1 polymorphic variants on DNA repair in cells exposed to X-rays. *Mutat. Res.* **2013**, *755*, 42–48. [CrossRef]
92. Mumbrekar, K.D.; Goutham, H.V.; Vadhiraja, B.M.; Bola Sadashiva, S.R. Polymorphisms in double strand break repair related genes influence radiosensitivity phenotype in lymphocytes from healthy individuals. *Dna Repair* **2016**, *40*, 27–34. [CrossRef]
93. Yin, M.; Liao, Z.; Huang, Y.J.; Liu, Z.; Yuan, X.; Gomez, D.; Wang, L.E.; Wei, Q. Polymorphisms of homologous recombination genes and clinical outcomes of non-small cell lung cancer patients treated with definitive radiotherapy. *PLoS ONE* **2011**, *6*, e20055. [CrossRef]
94. Venkatesh, G.H.; Manjunath, V.B.; Mumbrekar, K.D.; Negi, H.; Fernandes, D.J.; Sharan, K.; Banerjee, S.; Bola Sadashiva, S.R. Polymorphisms in radio-responsive genes and its association with acute toxicity among head and neck cancer patients. *PLoS ONE* **2014**, *9*, e89079. [CrossRef]
95. Chang-Claude, J.; Ambrosone, C.B.; Lilla, C.; Kropp, S.; Helmbold, I.; von Fournier, D.; Haase, W.; Sautter-Bihl, M.L.; Wenz, F.; Schmezer, P.; et al. Genetic polymorphisms in DNA repair and damage response genes and late normal tissue complications of radiotherapy for breast cancer. *Br. J. Cancer* **2009**, *100*, 1680–1686. [CrossRef] [PubMed]
96. Kerns, S.L.; Stock, R.G.; Stone, N.N.; Blacksburg, S.R.; Rath, L.; Vega, A.; Fachal, L.; Gómez-Caamaño, A.; De Ruysscher, D.; Lammering, G.; et al. Genome-wide association study identifies a region on chromosome 11q14.3 associated with late rectal bleeding following radiation therapy for prostate cancer. *Radiother. Oncol. J. Eur. Soc. Ther. Radiol. Oncol.* **2013**, *107*, 372–376. [CrossRef] [PubMed]

97. Ding, C.; Zhang, H.; Chen, K.; Zhao, C.; Gao, J. Genetic variability of DNA repair mechanisms influences treatment outcome of gastric cancer. *Oncol. Lett.* **2015**, *10*, 1997–2002. [CrossRef] [PubMed]
98. Erčulj, N.; Kovač, V.; Hmeljak, J.; Franko, A.; Dodič-Fikfak, M.; Dolžan, V. DNA repair polymorphisms and treatment outcomes of patients with malignant mesothelioma treated with gemcitabine-platinum combination chemotherapy. *J. Thorac. Oncol. Off. Publ. Int. Assoc. Study Lung Cancer* **2012**, *7*, 1609–1617. [CrossRef] [PubMed]
99. Ott, K.; Rachakonda, P.S.; Panzram, B.; Keller, G.; Lordick, F.; Becker, K.; Langer, R.; Buechler, M.; Hemminki, K.; Kumar, R. DNA repair gene and MTHFR gene polymorphisms as prognostic markers in locally advanced adenocarcinoma of the esophagus or stomach treated with cisplatin and 5-fluorouracil-based neoadjuvant chemotherapy. *Ann. Surg. Oncol.* **2011**, *18*, 2688–2698. [CrossRef]
100. Zhou, J.; Liu, Z.Y.; Li, C.B.; Gao, S.; Ding, L.H.; Wu, X.L.; Wang, Z.Y. Genetic polymorphisms of DNA repair pathways influence the response to chemotherapy and overall survival of gastric cancer. *Tumour Biol. J. Int. Soc. Oncodev. Biol. Med.* **2015**, *36*, 3017–3023. [CrossRef]
101. Jiang, Y.H.; Xu, X.L.; Ruan, H.H.; Xu, W.Z.; Li, D.; Feng, J.G.; Han, Q.B.; Mao, W.M. The impact of functional LIG4 polymorphism on platinum-based chemotherapy response and survival in non-small cell lung cancer. *Med. Oncol.* **2014**, *31*, 959. [CrossRef]
102. Sinitsky, M.Y.; Larionov, A.V.; Asanov, M.A.; Druzhinin, V.G. Associations of DNA-repair gene polymorphisms with a genetic susceptibility to ionizing radiation in residents of areas with high radon (222Rn) concentration. *Int. J. Radiat. Biol.* **2015**, *91*, 486–494. [CrossRef]
103. Senghore, T.; Wang, W.C.; Chien, H.T. Polymorphisms of Mismatch Repair Pathway Genes Predict Clinical Outcomes in Oral Squamous Cell Carcinoma Patients Receiving Adjuvant Concurrent Chemoradiotherapy. *Cancers* **2019**, *11*, 598. [CrossRef]
104. Dominguez-Valentin, M.; Drost, M.; Therkildsen, C.; Rambech, E.; Ehrencrona, H.; Angleys, M.; Lau Hansen, T.; de Wind, N.; Nilbert, M.; Juel Rasmussen, L. Functional implications of the p.Cys680Arg mutation in the MLH1 mismatch repair protein. *Mol. Genet. Genom. Med.* **2014**, *2*, 352–355. [CrossRef]
105. Dominguez-Valentin, M.; Wernhoff, P.; Cajal, A.R.; Kalfayan, P.G.; Piñero, T.A.; Gonzalez, M.L.; Ferro, A.; Sammartino, I.; Causada Calo, N.S.; Vaccaro, C.A. MLH1 Ile219Val Polymorphism in Argentinean Families with Suspected Lynch Syndrome. *Front. Oncol.* **2016**, *6*, 189. [CrossRef] [PubMed]
106. Blasi, M.F.; Ventura, I.; Aquilina, G.; Degan, P.; Bertario, L.; Bassi, C.; Radice, P.; Bignami, M. A human cell-based assay to evaluate the effects of alterations in the MLH1 mismatch repair gene. *Cancer Res.* **2006**, *66*, 9036–9044. [CrossRef] [PubMed]
107. Campbell, P.T.; Curtin, K.; Ulrich, C.M.; Samowitz, W.S.; Bigler, J.; Velicer, C.M.; Caan, B.; Potter, J.D.; Slattery, M.L. Mismatch repair polymorphisms and risk of colon cancer, tumour microsatellite instability and interactions with lifestyle factors. *Gut* **2009**, *58*, 661–667. [CrossRef] [PubMed]
108. Valentin, M.D.; Da Silva, F.C.; Santos, E.M.; Da Silva, S.D.; De Oliveira Ferreira, F.; Aguiar Junior, S.; Gomy, I.; Vaccaro, C.; Redal, M.A.; Della Valle, A.; et al. Evaluation of MLH1 I219V polymorphism in unrelated South American individuals suspected of having Lynch syndrome. *Anticancer Res.* **2012**, *32*, 4347–4351.
109. Nejda, N.; Iglesias, D.; Moreno Azcoita, M.; Medina Arana, V.; González-Aguilera, J.J.; Fernández-Peralta, A.M. A MLH1 polymorphism that increases cancer risk is associated with better outcome in sporadic colorectal cancer. *Cancer Genet. Cytogenet.* **2009**, *193*, 71–77. [CrossRef]
110. Li, S.; Zheng, Y.; Tian, T.; Wang, M.; Liu, X.; Liu, K.; Zhai, Y.; Dai, C.; Deng, Y.; Li, S.; et al. Pooling-analysis on hMLH1 polymorphisms and cancer risk: Evidence based on 31,484 cancer cases and 45,494 cancer-free controls. *Oncotarget* **2017**, *8*, 93063–93078. [CrossRef]
111. Zare, M.; Jafari-Nedooshan, J. Relevance of hMLH1 -93G>A, 655A>G and 1151T>A polymorphisms with colorectal cancer susceptibility: A meta-analysis based on 38 case-control studies. *Rev. Assoc. Med. Bras. (1992)* **2018**, *64*, 942–951. [CrossRef]
112. Zhang, Y.; Rohde, L.H.; Emami, K.; Hammond, D.; Casey, R.; Mehta, S.K.; Jeevarajan, A.S.; Pierson, D.L.; Wu, H. Suppressed expression of non-DSB repair genes inhibits gamma-radiation-induced cytogenetic repair and cell cycle arrest. *DNA Repair* **2008**, *7*, 1835–1845. [CrossRef]
113. Bakhtiari, E.; Monfared, A.S.; Niaki, H.A.; Borzoueisileh, S.; Niksirat, F.; Fattahi, S.; Monfared, M.K.; Gorji, K.E. The expression of MLH1 and MSH2 genes among inhabitants of high background radiation area of Ramsar, Iran. *J. Environ. Radioact.* **2019**, *208–209*, 106012. [CrossRef]

114. Yang, J.; Huang, Y.; Feng, Y.; Li, H.; Feng, T.; Chen, J.; Yin, L.; Wang, W.; Wang, S.; Liu, Y.; et al. Associations of Genetic Variations in Mismatch Repair Genes MSH3 and PMS1 with Acute Adverse Events and Survival in Patients with Rectal Cancer Receiving Postoperative Chemoradiotherapy. *Cancer Res. Treat. Off. J. Korean Cancer Assoc.* **2019**, *51*, 1198–1206. [CrossRef]
115. Miao, H.K.; Chen, L.P.; Cai, D.P.; Kong, W.J.; Xiao, L.; Lin, J. MSH3 rs26279 polymorphism increases cancer risk: A meta-analysis. *Int. J. Clin. Exp. Pathol.* **2015**, *8*, 11060–11067. [PubMed]
116. Ma, X.; Zhang, B.; Zheng, W. Genetic variants associated with colorectal cancer risk: Comprehensive research synopsis, meta-analysis, and epidemiological evidence. *Gut* **2014**, *63*, 326–336. [CrossRef] [PubMed]
117. Zhang, B.; Beeghly-Fadiel, A.; Long, J.; Zheng, W. Genetic variants associated with breast-cancer risk: Comprehensive research synopsis, meta-analysis, and epidemiological evidence. *Lancet Oncol.* **2011**, *12*, 477–488. [CrossRef]
118. Li, Z.; Pearlman, A.H.; Hsieh, P. DNA mismatch repair and the DNA damage response. *DNA Repair* **2016**, *38*, 94–101. [CrossRef]
119. Crouse, G.F. Non-canonical actions of mismatch repair. *DNA Repair* **2016**, *38*, 102–109. [CrossRef]
120. Conde, J.; Silva, S.N.; Azevedo, A.P.; Teixeira, V.; Pina, J.E.; Rueff, J.; Gaspar, J.F. Association of common variants in mismatch repair genes and breast cancer susceptibility: A multigene study. *BMC Cancer* **2009**, *9*, 344. [CrossRef]
121. Doherty, J.A.; Sakoda, L.C.; Loomis, M.M.; Barnett, M.J.; Julianto, L.; Thornquist, M.D.; Neuhouser, M.L.; Weiss, N.S.; Goodman, G.E.; Chen, C. DNA repair genotype and lung cancer risk in the beta-carotene and retinol efficacy trial. *Int. J. Mol. Epidemiol. Genet.* **2013**, *4*, 11–34.
122. Kappil, M.; Terry, M.B.; Delgado-Cruzata, L.; Liao, Y.; Santella, R.M. Mismatch Repair Polymorphisms as Markers of Breast Cancer Prevalence in the Breast Cancer Family Registry. *Anticancer Res.* **2016**, *36*, 4437–4441. [CrossRef]
123. Clark, N.; Wu, X.; Her, C. MutS Homologues hMSH4 and hMSH5: Genetic Variations, Functions, and Implications in Human Diseases. *Curr. Genom.* **2013**, *14*, 81–90. [CrossRef]
124. Chu, Y.L.; Wu, X.; Xu, J.; Watts, J.L.; Her, C. DNA damage induced MutS homologue hMSH4 acetylation. *Int. J. Mol. Sci.* **2013**, *14*, 20966–20982. [CrossRef]
125. He, Y.Z.; Chi, X.S.; Zhang, Y.C.; Deng, X.B.; Wang, J.R.; Lv, W.Y.; Zhou, Y.H.; Wang, Z.Q. NBS1 Glu185Gln polymorphism and cancer risk: Update on current evidence. *Tumour Biol. J. Int. Soc. Oncodev. Biol. Med.* **2014**, *35*, 675–687. [CrossRef] [PubMed]
126. Gao, P.; Ma, N.; Li, M.; Tian, Q.B.; Liu, D.W. Functional variants in NBS1 and cancer risk: Evidence from a meta-analysis of 60 publications with 111 individual studies. *Mutagenesis* **2013**, *28*, 683–697. [CrossRef] [PubMed]
127. Yao, F.; Fang, Y.; Chen, B.; Jin, F.; Wang, S. Association between the NBS1 Glu185Gln polymorphism and breast cancer risk: A meta-analysis. *Tumour Biol. J. Int. Soc. Oncodeve. Biol. Med.* **2013**, *34*, 1255–1262. [CrossRef] [PubMed]
128. Stern, M.C.; Lin, J.; Figueroa, J.D.; Kelsey, K.T.; Kiltie, A.E.; Yuan, J.M.; Matullo, G.; Fletcher, T.; Benhamou, S.; Taylor, J.A.; et al. Polymorphisms in DNA repair genes, smoking, and bladder cancer risk: Findings from the international consortium of bladder cancer. *Cancer Res.* **2009**, *69*, 6857–6864. [CrossRef]
129. Wang, J.; Liu, Q.; Yuan, S.; Xie, W.; Liu, Y.; Xiang, Y.; Wu, N.; Wu, L.; Ma, X.; Cai, T.; et al. Genetic predisposition to lung cancer: Comprehensive literature integration, meta-analysis, and multiple evidence assessment of candidate-gene association studies. *Sci. Rep.* **2017**, *7*, 8371. [CrossRef]
130. Wang, Y.; Sun, Z.; Xu, Y. Carriage of NBN polymorphisms and acute leukemia risk. *Int. J. Clin. Exp. Med.* **2015**, *8*, 3769–3776.
131. Zhang, Y.; Huang, Y.S.; Lin, W.Q.; Zhang, S.D.; Li, Q.W.; Hu, Y.Z.; Zheng, R.L.; Tang, T.; Li, X.Z.; Zheng, X.H. NBS1 Glu185Gln polymorphism and susceptibility to urinary system cancer: A meta-analysis. *Tumour Biol. J. Int. Soc. Oncodeve. Biol. Med.* **2014**, *35*, 10723–10729. [CrossRef]
132. Vineis, P.; Manuguerra, M.; Kavvoura, F.K.; Guarrera, S.; Allione, A.; Rosa, F.; Di Gregorio, A.; Polidoro, S.; Saletta, F.; Ioannidis, J.P.; et al. A field synopsis on low-penetrance variants in DNA repair genes and cancer susceptibility. *J. Natl. Cancer Inst.* **2009**, *101*, 24–36. [CrossRef]

133. Sud, A.; Hemminki, K.; Houlston, R.S. Candidate gene association studies and risk of Hodgkin lymphoma: A systematic review and meta-analysis. *Hematol. Oncol.* **2017**, *35*, 34–50. [CrossRef]
134. Mehdinejad, M.; Sobhan, M.R.; Mazaheri, M.; Zare Shehneh, M.; Neamatzadeh, H.; Kalantar, S.M. Genetic Association between ERCC2, NBN, RAD51 Gene Variants and Osteosarcoma Risk: A Systematic Review and Meta-Analysis. *Asian Pac. J. Cancer Prev. Apjcp* **2017**, *18*, 1315–1321. [CrossRef]

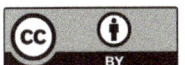

© 2020 by the authors. Licensee MDPI, Basel, Switzerland. This article is an open access article distributed under the terms and conditions of the Creative Commons Attribution (CC BY) license (http://creativecommons.org/licenses/by/4.0/).

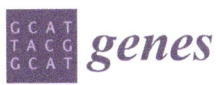

Review

Genetic Mutations and Variants in the Susceptibility of Familial Non-Medullary Thyroid Cancer

Fabíola Yukiko Miasaki [1], Cesar Seigi Fuziwara [2], Gisah Amaral de Carvalho [1] and Edna Teruko Kimura [2,*]

1. Department of Endocrinology and Metabolism (SEMPR), Hospital de Clínicas, Federal University of Paraná, Curitiba 80030-110, Brazil; fymiasaki@gmail.com (F.Y.M.); carvalho.gisah@gmail.com (G.A.d.C.)
2. Department of Cell and Developmental Biology, Institute of Biomedical Sciences, University of São Paulo, São Paulo 05508-000, Brazil; cesar.fuziwara@usp.br
* Correspondence: etkimura@usp.br; Tel.: +55-11-3091-7304

Received: 24 October 2020; Accepted: 16 November 2020; Published: 18 November 2020

Abstract: Thyroid cancer is the most frequent endocrine malignancy with the majority of cases derived from thyroid follicular cells and caused by sporadic mutations. However, when at least two or more first degree relatives present thyroid cancer, it is classified as familial non-medullary thyroid cancer (FNMTC) that may comprise 3–9% of all thyroid cancer. In this context, 5% of FNMTC are related to hereditary syndromes such as Cowden and Werner Syndromes, displaying specific genetic predisposition factors. On the other hand, the other 95% of cases are classified as non-syndromic FNMTC. Over the last 20 years, several candidate genes emerged in different studies of families worldwide. Nevertheless, the identification of a prevalent polymorphism or germinative mutation has not progressed in FNMTC. In this work, an overview of genetic alteration related to syndromic and non-syndromic FNMTC is presented.

Keywords: thyroid cancer; thyroid neoplasms; genetic predisposition to disease; genetic variants

1. Introduction

The most common type of thyroid cancer derives from thyroid follicular cells and is named as non-medullary thyroid cancer (NMTC) in order to be distinguished from the less frequent medullary thyroid cancer (MTC) that originates from the thyroid C-cells. The MTC occurs as sporadic and hereditary cancer, in contrast to the NMTC, which is mainly sporadic (Figure 1). The hereditary MTC can be a component of a syndrome or have a familial background. In this context, the NMTC can also be associated with syndromic conditions, such as in Cowden syndrome, Carney complex, Werner syndrome, and familial adenomatous polyposis but to a lesser extent than in MTC. Moreover, a high prevalence of NMTC in ataxia-telangiectasia, DICER1, and Pendred syndromes has been described [1,2].

Besides these well-known genetic syndromes, the characterization of the non-syndromic form of familial non-medullary thyroid cancer (FNMTC) remains to be consolidated. In 1953, Firminger and Skelton reported the first case of papillary thyroid cancer (PTC) in twins [3]. However, the concept of FNMTC and the genetic predisposition to PTC has emerged only in recent decades. Currently, it is accepted that FNMTC occurs when two or more first-degree relatives are diagnosed with NMTC cancer [4].

The initial FNMTC studies were performed by linkage analysis and described some specific loci, although they did not identify a precise gene associated with FMNTC [5–10]. Furthermore, despite the efforts of many groups in investigating FNMTC using Sanger sequencing, no conclusive information was found, suggesting genetic heterogeneity, multigenic inheritance, and multifactorial inheritance [11]. However, a new genomic perspective emerged with the application of Next Generation Sequencing

(NGS) technology that covered the entire genome. In this extent, some new insights into genetics of FNMTC have emerged by the recent genome-wide association studies (GWAS) in populations of PTC. The finding of several single nucleotide polymorphisms (SNPs), such as in *DIRC3*, *NIRG1*, *FOXE1*, *NKX2-1*, and *PCNXL2*, were observed in the European, Korean, and American populations [12]. Increasing evidence suggests that genetic predisposition factors play an essential role in carcinogenesis besides environmental factors [13]. In this review, we cover the genetic findings associated with FNMTC and in syndromes related to NMTC.

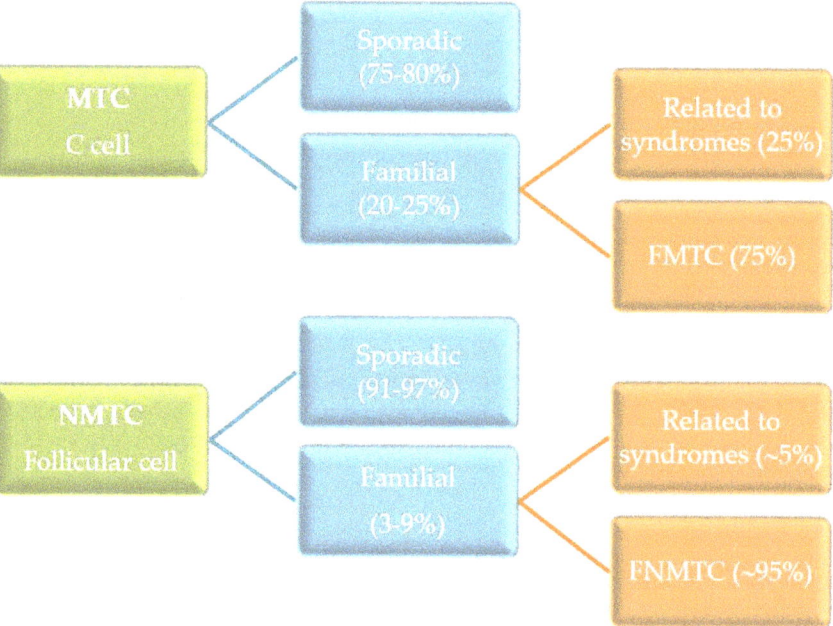

Figure 1. Incidence of sporadic and familial medullary thyroid cancer (MTC) and non-medullary thyroid cancer (NMTC).

2. Syndromic Causes of Non-Medullary Thyroid Cancer

Many syndromes associated with thyroid tumor predisposition have Mendelian patterns of inheritance, and they are related to mutations that may influence the mechanism of DNA repair, the microRNA processing, and maturation, the genome integrity maintenance, the cell signaling, or mitochondrial regulated cellular processes (Table 1) [13]. These syndromes are characterized by several other main malignancies and sometimes lack to present thyroid cancer. Some authors have suggested surveillance in syndromic FNMTC (see below). However, the guidelines, such as the 2015 American Thyroid Association's guideline, are precautious due to insufficient evidence in order to recommend the thyroid cancer screening [14].

Table 1. Genetic alterations in syndromes related to non-medullary thyroid cancer (NMTC).

Syndrome	Gene	Inheritance Pattern	Other Malignant Tumors	Prevalent Types of Thyroid Tumors	Benign Manifestations	Reference
Ataxia-telangiectasia syndrome *	ATM	AR *	Lymphocytic leukemia, lymphoma, stomach adenocarcinoma, medulloblastoma, glioma	FTC, PTC •	degenerative cerebellar atrophy, telangiectasias, immune defects	[15]
	ATM	AD	breast cancer, digestive tract cancer, lymphoma, leukemia			[15,16]
Carney complex	PRKAR1A	AD	-	Follicular hyperplasia, nodular hyperplasia, FA, cystic changes, PTC, FTC	Spotty skin pigmentation (lips, conjunctiva, vaginal, and penile mucosa), cutaneous and mucosal myxoma, cardiac myxoma, breast myxomatosis, primary pigmented nodular adrenocortical disease, GH-producing adenoma, large cell calcifying Sertoli cell tumors, psammomatous melanotic schwannomas	[17]
Cowden syndrome	PTEN, SDHB-D, SEC23B, KLLN, PARP4, AKT1, PIK3CA, USF3, TTN, RASAL1	AD	FTC, breast cancer, epithelial endometrial cancer, colon cancer, renal cell carcinoma melanoma	MNG, Hashimoto thyroiditis, FA, FTC, cPTC, FVPTC, C-cell hyperplasia	Macrocephaly	[18,19]
DICER1 syndrome	DICER1	AD	Pleuropulmonary blastoma, ovarian Sertoli-Leydig cell tumor, genitourinary and cerebral sarcomas	MNG, PTC, FA	MNG, cystic nephroma	[20,21]
Familial adenomatous polyposis	APC	AD	Digestive tract cancers, fibrosarcomas	CMVPTC, PTC	Intestinal polyps, osteomas, fibromas, desmoid tumors, dental abnormalities, leiomyomas, congenital hypertrophy of the retinal pigment epithelium	[22,23]
Li-Fraumeni syndrome	TP53	AD	Breast, brain, and adreno cortical cancers and sarcomas	cPTC, FVPTC		[13,24]
Werner syndrome	WRN	AR	Atypical melanoma, bone, or soft tissue sarcomas	FTC, PTC, ATC	Aging, bilateral cataract, type 2 diabetes mellitus, hypogonadism, meningioma	[2,25]

* Ataxia-telangiectasia syndrome occurs only in autosomal recessive pattern. However, heterozygotic carriers have an increased risk for thyroid cancer radio ionizing-induced. • An increased risk for thyroid cancer was observed in relatives of A-T patients, but the histological type was not specified in those epidemiological analysis. The above information is inferred from susceptibility thyroid cancer studies [26,27].

2.1. Cowden Syndrome

Cowden syndrome (OMIM #158350) is characterized by hamartomas in different parts of the body (gastrointestinal hamartomas, ganglioneuromas, trichilemmomas) associated with melanomas, breast, endometrial and thyroid cancer, macrocephaly, and, eventually, autism spectrum disorder and/or mental retardation [18,28]. One of the major diagnosis criteria is the presence of follicular thyroid carcinoma (FTC). However, if it is not detected, a biannual thyroid ultrasound is advocated in patients older than seven years [29].

Cowden syndrome is classically associated with mutations in the phosphatase and tensin homolog (*PTEN*) gene on chromosome 10q22–23, although variants in several other genes have been described in patients without *PTEN* mutations (*SDHB-D, SEC23B, KLLN, PARP4, AKT1, PIK3CA, USF3, TTN, MUTYH, RET, TSC2, BRCA1, BRCA2, ERCC2, HRAS*, and *RASAL1*) [19,30–32].

PTEN dephosphorylates PI (3,4,5) P3 (PIP3) and PI (3, 4) P2 to PI (4,5) P2 and PI (4) P, respectively. Thus, PIP3 and PI (3,4) P2 do not activate AKT serine/threonine kinase (AKT), and the phosphatidilinositol 3-kinase (PI3K)/AKT signaling pathway remains inhibited. PTEN mutation results in loss of function, leading to a high concentration of PI (3,4) P2 that activates AKT and enhances cell proliferation, cell migration, and reduces cell death [33,34]. In addition, mechanisms that regulate PTEN expression and compartmentalization are involved in tumorigenesis [35].

The first correlations between the PIK3-AKT pathway activation and thyroid cancer were observed in Cowden syndrome studies. Since Cowden syndrome mainly presents with FTC and PTEN activates the PIK3-AKT pathway, some authors have postulated that PIK3-AKT activation is required for FTC oncogenesis, and these preliminary findings were further corroborated [36,37].

Another intriguing fact was the association of RAS protein activator like 1 (*RASAL1*) with Cowden Syndrome. RASAL1 is a negative modulator of the RAS signaling pathway and suppresses both mitogen-activated protein kinase (MAPK) and PI3K pathways. However, *RASAL1* is frequently found methylated or mutated in sporadic follicular and anaplastic thyroid cancer [38].

In a large series of 155 patients with Cowden syndrome and thyroid cancer, 39 presented with *PTEN* germline mutations, while *RASAL1* germline alteration (*RASAL1*, c.982C>T, R328W) was observed in two patients without *PTEN* mutations [32]. In the same study, the authors also analyzed the germline database of The Cancer Genome Atlas (TCGA) and discovered that 0.6% of PTC patients harbored the deleterious germline *RASAL1* mutation [32].

2.2. Carney Complex

The Carney complex (OMIM #160980) is an autosomal dominant disorder in 70% of the cases, characterized by loss-of-function mutations in the *PRKAR1A* gene (17q22–24).

Under a normal condition of several endocrine related ligands, such as TSH, FSH, ACTH, GHRH, and MSH, when binding to the G-protein coupled receptor activates protein kinase A (PKA). *PRKAR1A* encodes the R1α subunit of PKA. Thus, when mutated, it increases cAMP-dependent PKA activity and drives tumorigenesis [17,39,40]. Therefore, thyrocytes, Sertoli cells, adrenocortical cells, somatotrophs, and melanocytes are directly affected by the *PRKAR1a* mutation. As a result, variable endocrine tumors are observed in the Carney complex disease, including primary pigmented nodular adrenocortical disease, pituitary adenomas, testicular tumors, ovarian lesions, and myxomas and lentiginosis syndromes [17]. Since thyroid cancer could also be part of this syndrome, annual long-term surveillance is recommended [17].

Evidence shows that PRKAR1A acts as a tumor suppressor gene in sporadic thyroid cancers [41]. However, the traditional thyroid cancer pathways (MAPK and PIK3-AKT pathways) are not involved in the Carney complex [42]. Instead, a recent in vitro study suggests that PKA activates AMP-activated kinase (AMPK) through serine/threonine kinase 11 (LKB1, also named SKT11) in Carney-related FTC without inhibiting mTOR activation [43].

2.3. Werner Syndrome

Werner syndrome is one of the progeroid syndromes (OMIM #27770) characterized by early aging, scleroderma-like skin changes, bilateral cataracts, and subcutaneous calcifications, premature arteriosclerosis, and diabetes mellitus. Different types of cancers are associated with this syndrome, such as meningiomas, myeloid disorders, soft tissue sarcomas, and thyroid carcinoma [1,44]. Their regular surveillance is recommended [45]. The Werner Syndrome's patients carry autosomal recessive WRN RecQ like helicase (*WRN*) gene mutations on 8p11.1–21.1. *WRN* gene encodes RecQ helicase that regulate DNA replication, recombination, repair, transcription, and telomerase maintenance. Dysregulation of this pathway triggers DNA instability, telomeric fusions of homologous chromosomes, and, ultimately, oncogenesis [13]. However, the precise mechanisms that contribute to genome instability in Werner syndrome remains unclear [46]. In a Japanese series, mutations in the N-terminal portion of *WRN* was correlated with PTC, while mutations in C-terminal with FTC [47]. The N-terminal portion of *WRN* contains exonuclease activity, whereas the central part contains the DNA-dependent ATPase, 3′–5′ helicase, and annealing activity [46]. Overall, these studies suggest specific effects in WRN activity depending on the site of mutation. Moreover, an in vitro study showed that mutations in *WRN*'s nuclease domain, helicase domain, or DNA binding domain aborted its canonical stimulatory effect on nonhomologous end-joining (c-NHEJ) pathway during DNA double-strand break (DSB) repair [46].

2.4. Familial Adenomatous Polyposis

The phenotype of familial adenomatous polyposis (FAP) (OMIM #175100) is characterized by numerous intestinal polyps, colon cancer, and other cancers that include thyroid cancer [2,22,48]. FAP is an autosomal dominant disorder caused by mutations in APC regulator of WNT signaling pathway (*APC*) gene on chromosome 5q21. The *APC* gene is a suppressor of the Wnt signaling pathway and regulates β-catenin activation by multiple mechanisms. In normal conditions, the Axin complex—formed by APC, glycogen synthase kinase 3 (GSK3), and casein kinase 1 (CK1)—phosphorylates the amino-terminal of the free β-catenin, permitting its recognition and further ubiquitination [49,50]. By this process of continuous degradation, β-catenin remains in the cytoplasm without reaching the promoter region of target genes in the nucleus. Thus, when the APC protein is mutated or truncated, β-catenin is released from its degradation and migrates to the nucleus, activating gene transcription of oncogenic pathways. Truncated APC protein also interferes with chromosome stability and cell migration [50].

In addition to the germline mutation, biallelic inactivation of the wild-type APC allele is frequently necessary for tumorigenesis, and the second-hit is commonly acquired by somatic mutation [51]. In the FAP-associated thyroid cancer, the concomitant presence of germline and distinct somatic mutation were observed in several Japanese families [48,52,53]. Most of FAP-associated thyroid cancers present the histological subtype called cribriform-morular variant of PTC (CMVPTC) [2,51]. An annual thyroid ultrasound is recommended to late teen years' patients [54,55].

2.5. Ataxia-Telangiectasia Syndrome

Ataxia-telangiectasia (A-T) syndrome (OMIM #208900) is an autosomal recessive disorder linked to the mutation of the ATM serine/threonine kinase (*ATM*) gene and characterized by degenerative cerebellar atrophy, telangiectasias, immune defects, and malignancy [56,57]. It is also well-known that relatives of patients with ataxia-telangiectasia have an increased cancer incidence [16].

ATM protein belongs to the PI-3 kinase-like protein kinases family. Besides TP53, BRCA1, and BRCA2, ATM is considered a genome's guardian and participates directly in the DNA damage response (DDR). For its activation, MRE11-RAD50-NBS1 (MRN) complex—A sensor of DSB (double strand-break)—induces several autophosphorylations and acetylations. Activated ATM then phosphorylates different proteins involved in the DSB (double-strand break) response [58].

For instance, ATM phosphorylates CHK2 and p53, which are both involved in senescence and apoptosis [58].

An increased incidence of thyroid cancer was observed in obligate *ATM* mutation carriers (RR adjusted = 2.6) [16]. Later, selective mutations in the *ATM* gene are related to thyroid cancer. *ATM* c.2119T>C p.S707P (rs4986761) heterozygotes were associated with an adjusted HR (hazard ratio for cancer) of 10 for thyroid/endocrine tumors, while no association was observed in *ATM* c.146C>G p.S49C (rs1800054) heterozygote carriers [56]. Nonetheless, recent population studies revealed that some ATM polymorphisms have a protective role, while other studies reported a damaging effect [59–62]. There are even controversial observations for the same polymorphism [26,27,59,60,63]. Despite these controversies, consistent *ATM* variants (*ATM* p.P1054R-rs1800057- and rs149711770) were recently described in families with FNMTC and other cancers (as kidney, lung, stomach, and prostate) [11]. Nonetheless, in A-T Syndrome's patient, the only screening recommended is for breast cancer [15].

2.6. DICER 1 Syndrome and miRNA Processing

A non-toxic multinodular goiter (MNG) is frequently diagnosed in the adult population and studies correlate the presence of MNG and the development of differentiated thyroid cancer [14,64,65]. On the other hand, familial cases of MNG are a common characteristic associated with the DICER1 syndrome (OMIM #601200), which predisposes patients to thyroid cancer [66], and other types of tumors such as Sertoli-Leydig cell tumors of the ovary (SLCT) [20] and pleuropulmonary blastomas [21].

DICER is an endonuclease essential for the maturation of microRNAs (miRNAs), small non-coding RNAs with ~22 nt, that block mRNA translation post-transcriptionally by binding to the 3'-UTR (untranslated region) of target mRNAs, and tightly controlling cell signaling and cell biology [67]. A mutation in dicer1, ribonuclease III (*DICER1*) gene, especially those present in the ribonuclease domain, leads to DICER loss of function and downregulation of microRNA levels [20,68]. The correct control of miRNA expression is essential for the development of a functional thyroid gland [69]. Studies with transgenic mice with dysfunctional DICER lead to disturbance of thyroid architecture, cell proliferation and disarrangement of follicular structures, and loss of differentiation [70,71], indicating the influence of DICER loss in thyroid tumorigenesis.

A familial approach to investigate the risk of thyroid malignancy in DICER1 syndrome patients revealed a 16-fold higher risk of development of thyroid cancer when *DICER1* is mutated compared to non-mutated patients [66]. Thus, there is a suggestion to monitor the thyroid status by a thyroid ultrasound every two-three years in patients after the age of eight [29,72]. Enforced evidence of *DICER1* mutation with familial thyroid cancer was also shown in a study with six individuals of the same family harboring *DICER1* mutation (c.5441C>T, p.S1814L) and multiple cases of differentiated thyroid cancer and MNG [73].

The Cancer Genome Atlas (TCGA) database shows *DICER1* mutation in 0.8% of patients with PTC/PDTC (p.E1813G, p.D1810H, p.E1813K, p.R1906S, p.M1402T) [74–78]. A recent study revealed high prevalence of *DICER1* mutations in pediatric-adolescent poorly differentiated thyroid cancer (83%) at a hotspot in the metal-ion binding sites of the RNase IIIb domain of DICER1 (c.5113G>A, p.E1705K, c.5125G>A, p.D1709N (rs1595331264), c.5137G>A, p.1713Y, c.5437G>A, p.E1813K, c.5437G>C, p.E1813Q) [79]. Another study linked hotspot *DICER1* mutations to pediatric PTC (c.5125G>A p.D1709N, c.5428G>T p.D1801Y, c.5438A>G p.E1813G, c.5439G>C p.E1813D) with increased incidence in the patients that do not harbor MAPK classic alterations [80], suggesting a role for *DICER1* mutation detection in thyroid tumors. A recent study detected *DICER1* (c.5429A>T, p.D1810V, c.5437G>A, p.E1813K) and drosha ribonuclease III (*DROSHA*) mutation (c.2943C>T, p.S981S, c.3597C>T, p.Y1199Y (rs61748189)) in benign follicular adenoma, even though *DICER1* mutations were not detected in a follicular variant of PTC that harbored *HRAS* mutations [68]. On the other hand, a recent study associated MAPK alterations with germline mutations in *DICER1* [81]. Altogether, these studies suggest that *DICER1* haploinsufficiency is associated with thyroid tumorigenesis.

DROSHA is another endonuclease of miRNA processing machinery and acts together with DGCR8 to form the Microprocessor complex to excise the precursor miRNA out of the primary transcript in the nucleus [67]. Then, DICER acts in the next step in the cytoplasm and cleaves the precursor miRNA to form mature functional miRNAs. In a similar extent to *DICER1* mutations, *DGCR8* mutations were also detected in familial cases of MNG and are associated with schwannoma [82]. Altogether, these studies indicate the essential role of proper miRNA processing and expression for thyroid gland physiology.

2.7. Li-Fraumeni Syndrome

The Li-Fraumeni syndrome is caused by a heterozygous mutation in *TP53* and is typically characterized by soft tissue and bone sarcomas, breast cancers, central nervous system tumors, leukemia, and adrenal tumors. p53 interacts with a complex network and drives DNA repair, cell-cycle arrest, senescence, or apoptosis when it is phosphorylated by DNA damage response (DDR) kinases [13,83]. The PTC occurs in 10% of Li-Fraumeni syndrome patients, mainly when associated with *TP53* mutation p.R337H [24]. Therefore, imaging screening for thyroid malignancy in Li-Fraumeni families has been advocated [24].

3. Non-Syndromic FNMTC

Even if FNMTC comprises only 3–9% of all thyroid cancer, the first-degree relatives of NMTC have an 8-12-fold increased risk of developing the disease [84,85]. Non-syndromic FNMTC comprises 95% of all FNMTC and is defined by two or more first-degree relatives present with NMTC without associated syndromes. Moreover, the transmission pattern is not yet well defined, which seems to be autosomal dominant in most cases. Like sporadic NMTC, more than 85% are PTC, approximately 10% are FTC, and around 5% are anaplastic thyroid cancer. Furthermore, FNMTC is more aggressive, presents with nodal disease, and recurs more often. In addition, thyroid cancer tends to occur earlier in subsequent generations in FNMTC, called the anticipation phenomenon [2,86,87].

3.1. Linkage Analysis

From 1997 to 2006, the linkage analysis was the main method to study the familial condition. Using this approach, a positive logarithm of odds (LOD) would mean a high likelihood that locus cosegregates with the FNMTC trait, which is a linkage. In this way, several loci were associated with non-syndromic FNMTC (Table 2).

Table 2. Loci and genes associated with non-syndromic familial non-medullary thyroid cancer (FNMTC).

Loci/Gene	Localization	Characteristics	Reference
Linkage analysis			
TCO	19p13.2	Oxyphilic PTC	[6]
NMTC1	2q21		[9]
PRN1	1q21	Papillary renal cancer	[8]
MNG1/*DICER1*	14q32	MNG	[7]
Linkage analysis and NGS			
SRGAP1	12q14		[88]
	8p23.1–p22		[10]
	6q22		[89]
lncRNA inside TG	8q24	Melanoma in 1 family	[90]
Enhancer associated with POU2F1 and YY1	4q32		[91]
Other methodology			
NKX2-1	14q13.3		[92]

3.1.1. TCO Locus (19p13.2)

The 'thyroid carcinoma, nonmedullary, with cell oxyphilia' (TCO) locus was identified in a French family with oxyphilic thyroid cancer in the short arm of chromosome 19 (19p13.2). This region includes several genes, such as *ICAM1* gene, which is overexpressed in thyroid cancer cells, and the JunB proto-oncogene, AP-1 transcription factor subunit (*JUNB*) [6]. However, some other genes in the locus, such as several zinc-finger-protein genes, were not yet identified. Moreover, the TCO locus does not seem to be involved in the majority of oxyphilic sporadic NMTC. An additional Tyrolean family with high LOD in the same locus was also described [93].

3.1.2. PRN1 Locus (1q21)

Papillary thyroid cancer is associated with papillary renal cancer. Linkage analysis identified this locus with the highest LOD of 3.58 in a family with three generations affected by PTC and papillary renal carcinoma. MET proto-oncogene, receptor tyrosine kinase (*MET*) mutations, frequently associated with familial papillary renal cancer, and mutations associated with other thyroid cancer syndromes were excluded [8]. However, this finding was limited to this family.

3.1.3. NMTC1 Locus (2q21)

This locus was described in a large Tasmanian family study [9], and when the authors further analyzed 17 families with FNMTC, they found an LOD heterogeneity of 4.17. At that time, it was hypothesized that multiple environmental and genetic causes could be involved in the pathogenesis of FNMTC [93].

3.1.4. q32 Locus (an Enhancer of Unknown Function)

A rare mutation in 4q32 was found in the linkage analysis and targeted deep sequencing in a large family with four individuals with benign thyroid disease, nine PTC patients, and one anaplastic thyroid cancer (ATC) patient. This nucleotide exchange in chr4:165491559 (GRCh37/hg19), named 4q32A>C, is in a highly conserved region. The chromatin immunoprecipitation (ChIP) assays showed that both POU2F1 and YY1 transcription factors related to specific thyroid genes and thyroid development bind to this region. As consequence of the allele's change, a decrease of both POUF2 and YY1 bindings were observed. Transcription factors' disruption has already been associated with cancer [91].

3.1.5. 6q22 Locus

The finding of 6q22 locus with LOD + 3.30 was observed in 38 families of FNMTC by linkage analysis and a genome-wide SNP array [89]. However, no further studies have confirmed this locus in additional families.

3.1.6. 8p23.1–p22 Locus

A locus associated with FNMTC in a huge Portuguese family was identified by linkage analysis, with a maximum parametric haplotype-based LOD score of 4.41. Among 17 candidate genes in the locus (*PPP1R3B, MIRN597, MIRN124A1, MSRA, C8orf74, SOX7, PINX1, MIRN598, C8orf15, C8orf16, MTMR9, C8orf13, NEIL2, CTSB, DUB3, DLC1, TUSC3*), no deleterious alteration was detected in the genes' coding region. [10].

3.1.7. 8q24 Locus, a lncRNA inside the Thyroglobulin (TG) Gene

Linkage analysis was also performed in a group of 26 families of PTC [90], which revealed a LOD of + 1.3 in a locus that harbors *TG* and *SLA* (Src like adaptor) genes. However, no polymorphism or mutation was found in the coding genes, suggesting that this alteration could be associated with a lncRNA related to the *TG* gene.

3.1.8. SRGAP1 (12q14 Locus)

The study of 38 families with FNMTC by genome-wide linkage analysis indicated a high peak in 12q14 in 55% (21 of 38), but with a modest OR = 1.21 (p = 0.0008). Nonetheless, it was observed six different germline mutations/variants in the *SRGAP1* gene (c.447A>C, p.Q149H, c.823G>A, p.A275T, c.1534G>A, p.V512I, rs74691643, c.1849C>T, p.R617C, rs114817817, c.2274T>C, p.S758S, rs789722, c.2624A>G, p.H875R, rs61754221). In vitro functional testing in thyroid cancer cells showed decreased GTPase activating protein (GAP) activity in two of these *SGARP1* polymorphisms (Q149H and R617C). The SRGAP1 could mediate tumorigenesis by interacting with CDC42 [88], which is a common signal transduction convergence point of many signaling pathways and can play a role in thyroid cancer cell migration via RAGE/Dia-1 signaling [94].

3.1.9. NKX2-1 (14q13.3 Locus)

The mutation in *NKX2-1* gene (c.1016 C>T, p. A339V) was described in two families associated with PTC and MNG [87]. Even though most patients had only MNG, the authors hypothesized that MNG could be the first step to malignancy [92,95–97].

3.1.10. MNG1 Locus (14q32)-DICER1

The MNG1 (OMIM # 138800) locus was revealed by linkage analysis in families with multinodular goiter and NMTC [7]. Furthermore, it was observed that MNG1 corresponded to *DICER1* gene, related to microRNA biogenesis (described in "Syndromic causes of non-medullary thyroid cancer" section).

3.2. Genome-Wide Linkage Analysis in the Population of PTC Patients

The sequencing of the genome by NGS uncovered the genetic variation and the potential association with several pathologies, including cancer. In particular, the GWAS (genome-wide association study) revealed numerous SNPs in the genes related to thyroid physiology and tumorigenesis (Table 3) [12].

Table 3. Genes associated with genetic predisposition of sporadic papillary thyroid cancer.

Locus	Nearest Gene	Population	Reference
9q22.33	FOXE1, PTCSC2	Belarus, Iceland, Italy, Korea, Netherlands Poland, Spain, USA	[98–100]
14q13.3	PTCSC3, NKX2-1, MBIP1	Iceland, Italy, Korea, Netherlands, Poland, Spain, USA	[98,99]
2q35	DIRC3	Iceland, Italy, Korea, Netherlands, Poland, Spain, UK, USA	[99,101]
8p12	NRG1	Iceland, Korea, Netherlands, Spain, USA	[99,102]
1q42.2	PCNXL2	Iceland, Korea, Netherlands, Spain, USA	[102,103]
European Only			
3q26.2	LRRC34	Iceland, Netherlands, Spain, USA	[103]
5p15.33	TERT	Iceland, Netherlands, Spain, USA	[103]
5q22.1	EPB41L4A	Iceland, Netherlands, Spain, USA	[103]
10q24.33	OBFC1	Iceland, Netherlands, Spain, USA	[103]
15q22.33	SMAD3	Iceland, Netherlands, Spain, USA	[103]
Korean Only			
12q14.3	MSRB3	Korea	[102]
1p13.3	VAV3	Korea	[102]
4q21.1	SEPT11	Korea	[102]
3p14.2	FHIT	Korea	[102]
19p13.2	INSR	Korea	[102]
12q24.13	SLC8B1	Korea	[102]

3.2.1. FOXE1/PTCSC2

Located in 9q22.3 and close to the forkhead box E1 (*FOXE1*) gene, rs965513 conferred an increased risk for thyroid cancer and was named 'papillary thyroid carcinoma susceptibility candidate 2' (*PTCSC2*) gene. The carriers of rs965513 (homozygous of A allele present a 3.1-fold increased risk for thyroid cancer in large European series [98]. The same polymorphism rs965513 was observed in Japanese and Belarusian populations, but with an OR of 1.6-1.9 [104]. Similarly, a variant in the promoter region of the *FOXE1* gene (rs1867277) was identified as a risk factor for PTC (OR = 1.49) in a Spanish series and further confirmed in an Italian one [105]. Subsequently, new studies showed a tumor suppressor effect of FOXE1 and demonstrated that rs1867277 is involved in differential recruitment of USF1/ USF2 transcription factors, which interferes with FOXE1 expression [12,106]. Moreover, myosin heavy chain-9 (MYH9) can bind and suppress the shared promoter of *PTCSC2* and *FOXE1* genes bilaterally (that includes rs1867277 region), an effect that is abolished by PTCSC2 that sequesters MYH9 [107]. Therefore, MYH9, which is a lncRNA binding protein, can also play a role in PTC susceptibility.

A rare *FOXE1* variant (c.743C>G; p.A248G) was identified in one of 60 Portuguese FNMTC cases and one sporadic case. Besides, polymorphisms in *FOXE1* locus (rs965513 and rs1867277) were associated with increased familial and sporadic NMTC risk [104,108].

3.2.2. NKX2-1

A consistent finding in the 14q13.3 locus was rs944289. Located close to the NKX2-1 gene, this variant of uncertain significance (VUS) is in PTCSC3's promoter region and regulates the lncRNA PTCSC3 expression by affecting the binding site of C/EBPα and C/EBPβ (PTCSC3 activators) [98,99,109,110]. PTCSC3 downregulates S100A4, reducing cell motility and invasiveness. Thus, *PTCSC3* mutations could predispose to PTC through the S100A4 pathway [111]. Moreover, *NKX2-1* mutation (c.1016C>T, p.A339V) was observed in a family with multinodular goiter and papillary thyroid cancer [87], but this was not confirmed by another FNMTC study [112].

3.2.3. NRG1

NRG1 polymorphisms produced an association signal in GWAS for thyroid cancer. NRG1 is highly expressed in the thyroid and participates in cell growth pathways, mainly via erb-b2 receptor tyrosine kinase (ERBB)/MAPK [113]. However, NRG1 expression is detected in follicular adenomas, suggesting they are linked to thyroid tumorigenesis [12].

3.2.4. DIRC3

Polymorphisms in the *DIRC3* (disrupted in renal carcinoma 3) gene have also been found in thyroid cancer GWAS [12,102,103]. *DIRC3* codifies a lncRNA that was first associated with renal cancer, suggesting a tumor suppressor role [101]. *DIRC3* and *IGFBP5* (insulin-like growth factor binding protein 5) tumor suppressors are within the same topologically associated domain. Moreover, it was observed that *DIRC3* depletion induces an increased *SOX10* (SRY-box transcription factor 10) repression of *IGFBP5* in melanoma cell cultures, corroborating the tumor suppressor role of *DIRC3* [114].

In addition, the TT variant of rs966423 (*DIRC3*, g.217445617C>T) has been associated with worse PTC presentation and prognosis. An increased tumor size, staging, lymph node involvement, and overall mortality was observed in the TT-haplotype [115]. In a Chinese series, rs966423 was also correlated to tumor invasion and multifocality [1]. Nevertheless, no difference in these parameters was observed in a Polish series [116].

3.2.5. Polygenic Contribution

Recently, an increased risk for PTC was associated with a cumulative number of deleterious polymorphisms detected in the same patient. Ten different polymorphisms (rs12129938, rs11693806, rs6793295, rs73227498, rs2466076, rs1588635, rs7902587, rs368187, rs116909374, and rs2289261) related to the PTC development were analyzed, and the presence of each of these SNPs increased the risk to PTC. Nevertheless, if a patient harbors all 10 variants at the same time, the risk of developing thyroid cancer is 6.9-fold greater than those with no variants [117].

3.2.6. Telomere Abnormalities

A decade ago, three independent groups observed that relative telomere length (RTL) is shorter in patients with FNMTC [118–120]. As telomerase controls the telomere length, one of these groups investigated *TERC* and *hTERT* (which form telomerase) alterations and observed the amplification of *hTERT* in patients' leukocytes [118]. However, this finding was not confirmed subsequently [119,120]. In recent years, many alterations in the shelterin complex's genes have been reported. The shelterin complex is formed by six proteins (POT1, ACD, TINF2, TERF1, TERF2, and TERF2IP), and protects the telomere from DDR mechanisms. Along with telomerase, this complex is vital for genomic stability because telomeric ends resemble DNA double breaks. Telomeric repeat binding factor 1 (TERF1, also known as TRF1), telomeric repeat binding factor 2 (TERF2, also known TRF2), and protection of telomeres 1 (POT1) directly recognize TTAGGG repeats. In contrast, adrenocortical dysplasia protein homolog (ACD, also known as TPP1), TERF1-interacting nuclear factor 2 (TINF2, also known as TIN2), and telomeric repeat binding factor 2 interacting protein (TERF2IP, also known as RAP1) form a complex that differentiates telomeres from sites of DNA damage.

TINF2 mutation was described in a family with melanoma and thyroid cancer predisposition. Functional analysis showed that mutated *TINF2* was unable to activate *TERF2*, resulting in longer telomere lengths. All shelterin complex's genes were screened in a subsequent 24 families with FNMTC, and two missense variants in *TINF2* and *ACD* genes were found, but only the *ACD* variant was predicted as deleterious [121].

Another group reported a new mutation in *POT1* (c.85G>T; p.V29L) [122] in an Italian FNMTC. *POT1* disruptions can interfere with the interaction of the POT1-ACD complex. In agreement with these findings, another *POT1* mutation (c.268A>G, p.K90E) was described in a family with a predisposition to several tumors (melanoma, breast, kidney, and thyroid cancer, pituitary tumor, and Cushing syndrome) [123]. Moreover, an association between the increased risk of thyroid cancer and the presence of an intronic variant of *POT1* (rs58722976) was also observed in a cohort of childhood cancer survivors [124].

Altogether, it suggests that telomere abnormalities and shelterin complex genes alteration may influence the predisposition to the FNMTC.

3.2.7. miRNA

The miRNA-related SNPs affect the microRNA biogenesis and function. A large study evaluated approximately 80 families displaying Mendelian-like inheritance and found two candidate miRNA (*let-7e* and *miR-181b*). The variants of let-7e and miR-182b-2 were located at the 5′ end of 3p mature miRNA and the 3′ end of 5p mature miRNA, respectively, which downregulate the expression by impairing the miRNA processing [125]. The gain or loss of specific miRNAs is an important oncogenic event [69].

3.3. Whole Exome/Genome Sequence

The whole-exome sequence (WES) or the whole genome sequence (WGS) of family members with FNMTC is another strategy besides the GWAS in large populations of differentiated thyroid cancer (DTC). Using this approach, an enormous number of variants is detected, demanding some criteria to filter and select the candidate variants. In general, minor allele frequency (MAF), the expression in thyroid and predictor functions (i.e., SIFT, PolyPhen, CADD, and others) are used as filters. Variants related to cancer pathways can also be used as filters. Since the application of this strategy has been consolidated for genetic studies in recent years, some authors have proposed new variants involved in FNMTC. Many are still under validation.

3.3.1. SRRM2

The association of linkage analysis and WES identified an *SRRM2* variant in a family with FNMTC [126]. However, this variant was not exclusively present in FNMTC, as it was found in sporadic NMTC cases, implying the occurrence of FNMTC may also depend on environmental factors or other genes [126].

3.3.2. NOP53

The presence of rs78530808 (*NOP53*, c.91G>C, p.D31H) was observed in one family with FNMTC when using a less strict filter than other studies (MAF < 2%) [116]. NOP53 participates in ribosome biogenesis and regulates the p53 activation in the case of ribosome biogenesis perturbation. The variant c.91G>C was also identified in three out of 44 families with FNMTC [127]. In the tumor samples, NOP53 expression was increased when compared to the adjacent normal tissue. Furthermore, NOP53 knockdown inhibited cell proliferation and colony formation in vitro [127]. Altogether, these findings suggested that this variant could have an oncogenic role in thyroid tumorigenesis [127].

3.3.3. HABP2

HABP2 variant is an excellent example to describe how careful we should be with possible false-positive findings. The variant G534E was described in a family with seven members with PTC [128]. However, this finding was severely criticized later by other researchers. Even though it seemed the right candidate in the beginning, further studies did not confirm it in other populations. Furthermore, since its MAF is high in the European population, we would expect a higher incidence of FNMTC [129]. Besides, the prevalence of this same variant was similar among patients with FNMTC, sporadic PTC, and controls [130,131].

3.4. Candidate Variants Associated with FNMTC

Recently, different groups have pinpointed a list of candidate variants in FNMTC. A Korean study identified seven candidate variants localized in *ANO7, CAV2, KANK1, PIK3CB, PKD1L1, PTPRF*, and *RHBDD2* genes in a family with four patients with PTC [132]. In addition, a Brazilian group reported seven new variants located in *FKBP10, PLEKHG5, P2RX5, SAPCD1, ANXA3, NTN4*, and *SERPINA1* [133].

In a large series including 17 families with isolated FNMTC and FNMTC associated with other malignancies, 41 rare candidate variants were identified in *TDRD6, IDE, TINF2, RNF213, AGK, NHLH1, TMCC1, ALB, THBS4, C5orf15, KLH3, FGFR4, SMARCD3, GPR107, NSMF, SVIL, EIF3, RNF169, NFRB, CIS, CDH11, EDC4, FOXA3, CDS2, NAPB, SALL4, ATG14, UNC79, LZTR1, ATP13A2, CTDSP1, MAPKAPK3, AARS, KDSR, ZNF302, ZNF17, ITGAD, FGD6, PDPR*, and *EFCAB8* genes. Cancer susceptibility genes (*CHEK2, PRF1, ATM, AKAP13, SLC26A11*) were also observed [11]. As described before, the authors further correlated the presence of *TINF2* (a shelterin gene) to families with PTC and melanoma.

It was also interesting to observe that some of these genes have already been associated with thyroid cancer predisposition [59,134]. Despite these promising findings, most of the variants need to be better investigated for its functional role in thyroid cancer risk.

4. Conclusions

It was expected that the advent of new technologies of genome study would shed new light on the genetic predisposition of FNMTC. The NGS certainly did shed light on a whole new spectrum of variants and pointed to the co-occurrence of several variants in FNMTC. However, the limiting point in this scenario is the lack of a detailed in vitro validation that could precisely identify the contribution of each variant for the complex FNMTC entity. Moreover, the expansion of already known genetic data in multiple cohorts is essential to establish their role in FNMTC carcinogenesis.

Author Contributions: E.T.K. conceived the idea; F.Y.M., C.S.F., G.A.d.C. and E.T.K. were involved in planning, writing, and editing the manuscript. All authors have read and agreed to the published version of the manuscript.

Funding: This study was financed in part by the CNPq (National Council for Scientific and Technological Development-Brazil) grant 430756/2018-6 (E.T.K.).

Acknowledgments: We gratefully acknowledge the CNPq by the grant 308331/2017-6 (E.T.K.), FAPESP (The São Paulo Research Foundation-Brazil) by the grant 2020/10403-9 (C.S.F.), and the scholarships from CAPES (Coordenação de Aperfeiçoamento de Pessoal de Nível Superior-Brazil): PDSE 88881.362254/2019-01 (F.Y.M.) and PNPD 88887.374682/2019-00 (C.S.F.).

Conflicts of Interest: The authors declare no conflict of interest.

Abbreviations

AD	autosomal dominant
AR	autosomal recessive
ATC	anaplastic thyroid cancer
CMVPTC	cribriform-morular variant of PTC
cPTC	classical PTC
DDR	DNA damage response
DTC	differentiated thyroid cancer
FA	follicular adenoma
FAP	familial adenomatous polyposis
FNMTC	familial nonmedullary thyroid cancer
FTC	follicular thyroid cancer
FVPTC	follicular variant of PTC
GWAS	genome-wide association studies
HR	hazard ratio
LOD	logarithm of odds
MAF	minor allele frequency
miRNAs	microRNAs
MNG	multinodular goiter
MTC	medullary thyroid cancer
NGS	next generation sequencing
NMTC	nonmedullary thyroid cancer
PTC	papillary thyroid cancer
SNPs	single nucleotide polymorphisms
TCGA	The Cancer Genome Atlas
VUS	variant of uncertain significance
WES	whole exome sequence
WGS	whole genome sequence

References

1. Hincza, K.; Kowalik, A.; Kowalska, A. Current Knowledge of Germline Genetic Risk Factors for the Development of Non-Medullary Thyroid Cancer. *Genes* **2019**, *10*, 482. [CrossRef] [PubMed]
2. Guilmette, J.; Nosé, V. Hereditary and familial thyroid tumours. *Histopathology* **2017**, *72*, 70–81. [CrossRef] [PubMed]
3. Firminger, H.I.; Skelton, F.R. Carcinoma of the thyroid: Papillary adenocarcinoma occurring in twins and a case of Hürthle cell carcinoma; tumor conference. *J. Kans. Med. Soc.* **1953**, *54*, 427–432. [PubMed]
4. Sippel, R.S.; Caron, N.R.; Clark, O.H. An evidence-based approach to familial nonmedullary thyroid cancer: Screening, clinical management, and follow-up. *World J. Surg.* **2007**, *31*, 924–933. [CrossRef] [PubMed]

5. Mazeh, H.; Sippel, R.S. Familial nonmedullary thyroid carcinoma. *Thyroid* **2013**, *23*, 1049–1056. [CrossRef]
6. Canzian, F.; Amati, P.; Harach, H.R.; Kraimps, J.-L.; Lesueur, F.; Barbier, J.; Levillain, P.; Romeo, G.; Bonneau, D. A gene predisposing to familial thyroid tumors with cell oxyphilia maps to chromosome 19p13.2. *Am. J. Hum. Genet.* **1998**, *63*, 1743–1748. [CrossRef]
7. Bignell, G.R.; Canzian, F.; Shayeghi, M.; Stark, M.; Shugart, Y.Y.; Biggs, P.; Mangion, J.; Hamoudi, R.; Rosenblatt, J.; Buu, P.; et al. Familial nontoxic multinodular thyroid goiter locus maps to chromosome 14q but does not account for familial nonmedullary thyroid cancer. *Am. J. Hum. Genet.* **1997**, *61*, 1123–1130. [CrossRef]
8. Malchoff, C.D.; Sarfarazi, M.; Tendler, B.; Forouhar, F.; Whalen, G.; Joshi, V.; Arnold, A.; Malchoff, D.M. Papillary thyroid carcinoma associated with papillary renal neoplasia: Genetic linkage analysis of a distinct heritable tumor syndrome. *J. Clin. Endocrinol. Metab.* **2000**, *85*, 1758–1764. [CrossRef]
9. McKay, J.D.; Lesueur, F.; Jonard, L.; Pastore, A.; Williamson, J.; Hoffman, L.; Burgess, J.; Duffield, A.; Papotti, M.; Stark, M.; et al. Localization of a susceptibility gene for familial nonmedullary thyroid carcinoma to chromosome 2q21. *Am. J. Hum. Genet.* **2001**, *69*, 440–446. [CrossRef]
10. Cavaco, B.M.; Batista, P.F.; Sobrinho, L.G.; Leite, V. Mapping a new familial thyroid epithelial neoplasia susceptibility locus to chromosome 8p23.1-p22 by high-density single-nucleotide polymorphism genome-wide linkage analysis. *J. Clin. Endocrinol. Metab.* **2008**, *93*, 4426–4430. [CrossRef]
11. Wang, Y.; Liyanarachchi, S.; Miller, K.E.; Nieminen, T.T.; Comiskey, D.F., Jr.; Li, W.; Brock, P.; Symer, D.E.; Akagi, K.; DeLap, K.E.; et al. Identification of Rare Variants Predisposing to Thyroid Cancer. *Thyroid* **2019**, *29*, 946–955. [CrossRef] [PubMed]
12. Saenko, V.A.; Rogounovitch, T.I. Genetic Polymorphism Predisposing to Differentiated Thyroid Cancer: A Review of Major Findings of the Genome-Wide Association Studies. *Endocrinol. Metab.* **2018**, *33*, 164–174. [CrossRef]
13. Carbone, M.; Arron, S.T.; Beutler, B.; Bononi, A.; Cavenee, W.; Cleaver, J.E.; Croce, C.M.; D'Andrea, A.; Foulkes, W.D.; Gaudino, G.; et al. Tumour predisposition and cancer syndromes as models to study gene-environment interactions. *Nat. Rev. Cancer* **2020**, *20*, 533–549. [CrossRef] [PubMed]
14. Haugen, B.R.; Alexander, E.K.; Bible, K.C.; Doherty, G.M.; Mandel, S.J.; Nikiforov, Y.E.; Pacini, F.; Randolph, G.W.; Sawka, A.M.; Schlumberger, M.; et al. 2015 American Thyroid Association Management Guidelines for Adult Patients with Thyroid Nodules and Differentiated Thyroid Cancer: The American Thyroid Association Guidelines Task Force on Thyroid Nodules and Differentiated Thyroid Cancer. *Thyroid* **2016**, *26*, 1–133. [CrossRef]
15. Van Os, N.J.; Roeleveld, N.; Weemaes, C.M.R.; Jongmans, M.C.J.; Janssens, G.O.; Taylor, A.M.R.; Hoogerbrugge, N.; Willemsen, M.A.A.P. Health risks for ataxia-telangiectasia mutated heterozygotes: A systematic review, meta-analysis and evidence-based guideline. *Clin. Genet.* **2016**, *90*, 105–117. [CrossRef] [PubMed]
16. Geoffroy-Perez, B.; Janin, N.; Ossian, K.; Laugé, A.; Croquette, M.F.; Griscelli, C.; Debré, M.; Bressac-de-Paillerets, B.; Aurias, A.; Stoppa-Lyonnet, D.; et al. Cancer risk in heterozygotes for ataxia-telangiectasia. *Int. J. Cancer* **2001**, *93*, 288–293. [CrossRef]
17. Kamilaris, C.D.C.; Faucz, F.R.; Voutetakis, A.; Stratakis, C.A. Carney Complex. *Exp. Clin. Endocrinol. Diabetes* **2019**, *127*, 156–164. [CrossRef]
18. Gammon, A.; Jasperson, K.; Champine, M. Genetic basis of Cowden syndrome and its implications for clinical practice and risk management. *Appl. Clin. Genet.* **2016**, *9*, 83–92. [CrossRef]
19. Yehia, L.; Keel, E.; Eng, C. The Clinical Spectrum of PTEN Mutations. *Annu. Rev. Med.* **2020**, *71*, 103–116. [CrossRef]
20. Frio, T.R.; Bahubeshi, A.; Kanellopoulou, C.; Hamel, N.; Niedziela, M.; Sabbaghian, N.; Pouchet, C.; Gilbert, L.; O'Brien, P.K.; Serfas, K.; et al. DICER1 Mutations in Familial Multinodular Goiter With and Without Ovarian Sertoli-Leydig Cell Tumors. *JAMA* **2011**, *305*, 68–77. [CrossRef]
21. Hill, D.A.; Ivanovich, J.; Priest, J.R.; Gurnett, C.A.; Dehner, L.P.; Desruisseau, D.; Jarzembowski, J.A.; Wikenheiser-Brokamp, K.A.; Suarez, B.K.; Whelan, A.J.; et al. DICER1 Mutations in Familial Pleuropulmonary Blastoma. *Science* **2009**, *325*, 965. [CrossRef] [PubMed]
22. Tomoda, C.; Miyauchi, A.; Uruno, T.; Takamura, Y.; Ito, Y.; Miya, A.; Kobayashi, K.; Matsuzuka, F.; Kuma, S.; Kuma, K.; et al. Cribriform-morular variant of papillary thyroid carcinoma: Clue to early detection of familial adenomatous polyposis-associated colon cancer. *World J. Surg.* **2004**, *28*, 886–889. [CrossRef] [PubMed]

23. Nieminen, T.T.; Walker, C.J.; Olkinuora, A.; Genutis, L.K.; O'Malley, M.; Wakely, P.E.; LaGuardia, L.; Koskenvuo, L.; Arola, J.; Lepistö, A.H.; et al. Thyroid Carcinomas That Occur in Familial Adenomatous Polyposis Patients Recurrently Harbor Somatic Variants in APC, BRAF, and KTM2D. *Thyroid* **2020**, *30*, 380–388. [CrossRef] [PubMed]
24. Formiga, M.N.D.C.; De Andrade, K.C.; Kowalski, L.P.; Achatz, M.I. Frequency of Thyroid Carcinoma in Brazilian TP53 p.R337H Carriers with Li Fraumeni Syndrome. *JAMA Oncol.* **2017**, *3*, 1400–1402. [CrossRef] [PubMed]
25. Oshima, J.; Sidorova, J.M.; Monnat, R.J., Jr. Werner syndrome: Clinical features, pathogenesis and potential therapeutic interventions. *Ageing Res. Rev.* **2017**, *33*, 105–114. [CrossRef] [PubMed]
26. Pereda, C.M.; Lesueur, F.; Pertesi, M.; Robinot, N.; Lence-Anta, J.J.; Turcios, S.; Velasco, M.; Chappe, M.; Infante, I.; Bustillo, M.; et al. Common variants at the 9q22.33, 14q13.3 and ATM loci, and risk of differentiated thyroid cancer in the Cuban population. *BMC Genet.* **2015**, *16*, 22. [CrossRef]
27. Maillard, S.; Damiola, F.; Clero, E.; Pertesi, M.; Robinot, N.; Rachédi, F.; Boissin, J.-L.; Sebbag, J.; Shan, L.; Bost-Bezeaud, F.; et al. Common variants at 9q22.33, 14q13.3, and ATM loci, and risk of differentiated thyroid cancer in the French Polynesian population. *PLoS ONE* **2015**, *10*, e0123700. [CrossRef]
28. Tan, M.-H.; Mester, J.; Peterson, C.; Yang, Y.; Chen, J.-L.; Rybicki, L.A.; Milas, K.; Pederson, H.; Remzi, B.; Orloff, M.S.; et al. A clinical scoring system for selection of patients for PTEN mutation testing is proposed on the basis of a prospective study of 3042 probands. *Am. J. Hum. Genet.* **2011**, *88*, 42–56. [CrossRef]
29. Schultz, K.A.P.; Rednam, S.P.; Kamihara, J.; Doros, L.; Achatz, M.I.; Wasserman, J.D.; Diller, L.R.; Brugières, L.; Druker, H.; Schneider, K.A.; et al. PTEN, DICER1, FH, and Their Associated Tumor Susceptibility Syndromes: Clinical Features, Genetics, and Surveillance Recommendations in Childhood. *Clin. Cancer Res.* **2017**, *23*, e76–e82. [CrossRef]
30. Ikeda, Y.; Kiyotani, K.; Yew, P.Y.; Kato, T.; Tamura, K.; Yap, K.L.; Nielsen, S.M.; Mester, J.L.; Eng, C.; Nakamura, Y.; et al. Germline PARP4 mutations in patients with primary thyroid and breast cancers. *Endocr. Relat. Cancer* **2016**, *23*, 171–179. [CrossRef]
31. Yehia, L.; Ni, Y.; Sesock, K.; Niazi, F.; Fletcher, B.; Chen, H.J.L.; LaFramboise, T.; Eng, C. Unexpected cancer-predisposition gene variants in Cowden syndrome and Bannayan-Riley-Ruvalcaba syndrome patients without underlying germline PTEN mutations. *PLoS Genet.* **2018**, *14*, e1007352. [CrossRef] [PubMed]
32. Ngeow, J.; Ni, Y.; Tohme, R.; Chen, F.S.; Bebek, G.; Eng, C. Germline alterations in RASAL1 in Cowden syndrome patients presenting with follicular thyroid cancer and in individuals with apparently sporadic epithelial thyroid cancer. *J. Clin. Endocrinol. Metab.* **2014**, *99*, E1316–E1321. [CrossRef] [PubMed]
33. Naderali, E.; Khaki, A.A.; Rad, J.S.; Ali-Hemmati, A.; Rahmati, M.; Charoudeh, H.N. Regulation and modulation of PTEN activity. *Mol. Biol. Rep.* **2018**, *45*, 2869–2881. [CrossRef] [PubMed]
34. Costa, H.A.; Leitner, M.G.; Sos, M.L.; Mavrantoni, A.; Rychkova, A.; Johnson, J.R.; Newton, B.W.; Yee, M.C.; De La Vega, F.M.; Ford, J.M.; et al. Discovery and functional characterization of a neomorphic PTEN mutation. *Proc. Natl. Acad. Sci. USA* **2015**, *112*, 13976–13981. [CrossRef] [PubMed]
35. Milella, M.; Falcone, I.; Conciatori, F.; Cesta Incani, U.; Del Curatolo, A.; Inzerilli, N.; Nuzzo, C.M.; Vaccaro, V.; Vari, S.; Cognetti, F.; et al. PTEN: Multiple Functions in Human Malignant Tumors. *Front. Oncol.* **2015**, *5*, 24. [CrossRef]
36. Ringel, M.D.; Hayre, N.; Saito, J.; Saunier, B.; Schuppert, F.; Burch, H.; Bernet, V.; Burman, K.D.; Kohn, L.D.; Saji, M. Overexpression and overactivation of Akt in thyroid carcinoma. *Cancer Res.* **2001**, *61*, 6105–6111.
37. Xing, M. Molecular pathogenesis and mechanisms of thyroid cancer. *Nat. Rev. Cancer* **2013**, *13*, 184–199. [CrossRef]
38. Liu, D.; Yang, C.; Bojdani, E.; Murugan, A.K.; Xing, M. Identification of RASAL1 as a major tumor suppressor gene in thyroid cancer. *J. Natl. Cancer Inst.* **2013**, *105*, 1617–1627. [CrossRef]
39. Pepe, S.; Korbonits, M.; Iacovazzo, D. Germline and mosaic mutations causing pituitary tumours: Genetic and molecular aspects. *J. Endocrinol.* **2019**, *240*, R21–R45. [CrossRef]
40. Griffin, K.J.; Kirschner, L.S.; Matyakhina, L.; Stergiopoulos, S.; Robinson-White, A.; Lenherr, S.; Weinberg, F.D.; Claflin, E.; Meoli, E.; Cho-Chung, Y.S.; et al. Down-regulation of regulatory subunit type 1A of protein kinase A leads to endocrine and other tumors. *Cancer Res.* **2004**, *64*, 8811–8815. [CrossRef]
41. Sandrini, F.; Matyakhina, L.; Sarlis, N.J.; Kirschner, L.S.; Farmakidis, C.; Gimm, O.; Stratakis, C.A. Regulatory subunit type I-α of protein kinase A (PRKAR1A): A tumor-suppressor gene for sporadic thyroid cancer. *Genes Chromosomes Cancer* **2002**, *35*, 182–192. [CrossRef] [PubMed]

42. Pringle, D.R.; Yin, Z.; Lee, A.A.; Manchanda, P.K.; Yu, L.; Parlow, A.F.; Jarjoura, D.; La Perle, K.M.D.; Kirschner, L.S. Thyroid-specific ablation of the Carney complex gene, PRKAR1A, results in hyperthyroidism and follicular thyroid cancer. *Endocrine-Related Cancer* **2012**, *19*, 435–446. [CrossRef] [PubMed]
43. Kari, S.; Vasko, V.V.; Priya, S.; Kirschner, L.S. PKA Activates AMPK Through LKB1 Signaling in Follicular Thyroid Cancer. *Front. Endocrinol.* **2019**, *10*, 769. [CrossRef] [PubMed]
44. Goto, M.; Miller, R.W.; Ishikawa, Y.; Sugano, H. Excess of rare cancers in Werner syndrome (adult progeria). *Cancer Epidemiol. Biomarkers Prev.* **1996**, *5*, 239–246. [PubMed]
45. Muftuoglu, M.; Oshima, J.; von Kobbe, C.; Cheng, W.H.; Leistritz, D.F.; Bohr, V.A. The clinical characteristics of Werner syndrome: Molecular and biochemical diagnosis. *Hum. Genet.* **2008**, *124*, 369–377. [CrossRef]
46. Shamanna, R.A.; Lu, H.; de Freitas, J.K.; Tian, J.; Croteau, D.L.; Bohr, V.A. WRN regulates pathway choice between classical and alternative non-homologous end joining. *Nat. Commun.* **2016**, *7*, 13785. [CrossRef]
47. Ishikawa, Y.; Sugano, H.; Matsumoto, T.; Furuichi, Y.; Miller, R.W.; Goto, M. Unusual features of thyroid carcinomas in Japanese patients with Werner syndrome and possible genotype-phenotype relations to cell type and race. *Cancer* **1999**, *85*, 1345–1352. [CrossRef]
48. Uchino, S.; Noguchi, S.; Yamashita, H.; Yamashita, H.; Watanabe, S.; Ogawa, T.; Tsuno, A.; Murakami, A.; Miyauchi, A. Mutational analysis of the APC gene in cribriform-morula variant of papillary thyroid carcinoma. *World J. Surg.* **2006**, *30*, 775–779. [CrossRef]
49. De Herreros, A.G.; Duñach, M. Intracellular Signals Activated by Canonical Wnt Ligands Independent of GSK3 Inhibition and β-Catenin Stabilization. *Cells* **2019**, *8*, 1148. [CrossRef]
50. Heinen, C.D. Genotype to phenotype: Analyzing the effects of inherited mutations in colorectal cancer families. *Mutat. Res.* **2010**, *693*, 32–45. [CrossRef]
51. Giannelli, S.M.; McPhaul, L.; Nakamoto, J.; Gianoukakis, A.G. Familial adenomatous polyposis-associated, cribriform morular variant of papillary thyroid carcinoma harboring a K-RAS mutation: Case presentation and review of molecular mechanisms. *Thyroid* **2014**, *24*, 1184–1189. [CrossRef]
52. Iwama, T.; Konishi, M.; Iijima, T.; Yoshinaga, K.; Tominaga, T.; Koike, M.; Miyaki, M. Somatic mutation of the APC gene in thyroid carcinoma associated with familial adenomatous polyposis. *Jpn. J. Cancer Res.* **1999**, *90*, 372–376. [CrossRef] [PubMed]
53. Miyaki, M.; Iijima, T.; Ishii, R.; Hishima, T.; Mori, T.; Yoshinaga, K.; Takami, H.; Kuroki, T.; Iwama, T. Molecular Evidence for Multicentric Development of Thyroid Carcinomas in Patients with Familial Adenomatous Polyposis. *Am. J. Pathol.* **2000**, *157*, 1825–1827. [CrossRef]
54. Syngal, S.; Brand, R.E.; Church, J.M.; Giardiello, F.M.; Hampel, H.L.; Burt, R.W. ACG clinical guideline: Genetic testing and management of hereditary gastrointestinal cancer syndromes. *Am. J. Gastroenterol.* **2015**, *110*, 223–262. [CrossRef] [PubMed]
55. Achatz, M.I.; Porter, C.C.; Brugières, L.; Druker, H.; Frebourg, T.; Foulkes, W.D.; Kratz, C.P.; Kuiper, R.P.; Hansford, J.R.; Hernandez, H.S.; et al. Cancer Screening Recommendations and Clinical Management of Inherited Gastrointestinal Cancer Syndromes in Childhood. *Clin. Cancer Res.* **2017**, *23*, e107–e114. [CrossRef]
56. Dombernowsky, S.L.; Weischer, M.; Allin, K.H.; Bojesen, S.E.; Tybjirg-Hansen, A.; Nordestgaard, B.G. Risk of cancer by ATM missense mutations in the general population. *J. Clin. Oncol.* **2008**, *26*, 3057–3062. [CrossRef]
57. Shiloh, Y. ATM: Expanding roles as a chief guardian of genome stability. *Exp. Cell Res.* **2014**, *329*, 154–161. [CrossRef]
58. Ribezzo, F.; Shiloh, Y.; Schumacher, B. Systemic DNA damage responses in aging and diseases. *Semin. Cancer Biol.* **2016**, *37–38*, 26–35. [CrossRef]
59. Akulevich, N.M.; Saenko, V.A.; Rogounovitch, T.I.; Drozd, V.M.; Lushnikov, E.F.; Ivanov, V.K.; Mitsutake, N.; Kominami, R.; Yamashita, S. Polymorphisms of DNA damage response genes in radiation-related and sporadic papillary thyroid carcinoma. *Endocr. Relat. Cancer* **2009**, *16*, 491–503. [CrossRef]
60. Xu, L.; Morari, E.C.; Wei, Q.; Sturgis, E.M.; Ward, L.S. Functional variations in the ATM gene and susceptibility to differentiated thyroid carcinoma. *J. Clin. Endocrinol. Metab.* **2012**, *97*, 1913–1921. [CrossRef]
61. Gu, Y.; Shi, J.; Qiu, S.; Qiao, Y.; Zhang, X.; Cheng, Y.; Liu, Y. Association between ATM rs1801516 polymorphism and cancer susceptibility: A meta-analysis involving 12,879 cases and 18,054 controls. *BMC Cancer* **2018**, *18*, 1060. [CrossRef]

62. Song, C.M.; Kwon, T.K.; Park, B.L.; Ji, Y.B.; Tae, K. Single nucleotide polymorphisms of ataxia telangiectasia mutated and the risk of papillary thyroid carcinoma. *Environ. Mol. Mutagen.* **2015**, *56*, 70–76. [CrossRef] [PubMed]
63. Wójcicka, A.; Czetwertyńska, M.; Świerniak, M.; Długosińska, J.; Maciąg, M.; Czajka, A.; Dymecka, K.; Kubiak, A.; Kot, A.; Płoski, R.; et al. Variants in the ATM-CHEK2-BRCA1 axis determine genetic predisposition and clinical presentation of papillary thyroid carcinoma. *Genes Chromosomes Cancer* **2014**, *53*, 516–523. [CrossRef] [PubMed]
64. Kitahara, C.M.; Farkas, D.K.R.; Jørgensen, J.O.L.; Cronin-Fenton, D.; Sørensen, H.T. Benign Thyroid Diseases and Risk of Thyroid Cancer: A Nationwide Cohort Study. *J. Clin. Endocrinol. Metab.* **2018**, *103*, 2216–2224. [CrossRef] [PubMed]
65. Smith, J.J.; Chen, X.; Schneider, D.F.; Broome, J.T.; Sippel, R.S.; Chen, H.; Solórzano, C.C. Cancer after Thyroidectomy: A Multi-Institutional Experience with 1,523 Patients. *J. Am. Coll. Surg.* **2013**, *216*, 571–577. [CrossRef] [PubMed]
66. Khan, N.E.; Bauer, A.J.; Schultz, K.A.P.; Doros, L.; DeCastro, R.M.; Ling, A.; Lodish, M.B.; Harney, L.A.; Kase, R.G.; Carr, A.G.; et al. Quantification of Thyroid Cancer and Multinodular Goiter Risk in the DICER1 Syndrome: A Family-Based Cohort Study. *J. Clin. Endocrinol. Metab.* **2017**, *102*, 1614–1622. [CrossRef]
67. Lin, S.; Gregory, R.I. MicroRNA biogenesis pathways in cancer. *Nat. Rev. Cancer* **2015**, *15*, 321–333. [CrossRef]
68. Poma, A.M.; Condello, V.; Denaro, M.; Torregrossa, L.; Elisei, R.; Vitti, P.; Basolo, F. DICER1 somatic mutations strongly impair miRNA processing even in benign thyroid lesions. *Oncotarget* **2019**, *10*, 1785–1797. [CrossRef]
69. Fuziwara, C.S.; Kimura, E.T. MicroRNAs in thyroid development, function and tumorigenesis. *Mol. Cell. Endocrinol.* **2017**, *456*, 44–50. [CrossRef]
70. Rodriguez, W.; Jin, L.; Janssens, V.; Pierreux, C.; Hick, A.-C.; Urizar, E.; Costagliola, S. Deletion of the RNaseIII Enzyme Dicer in Thyroid Follicular Cells Causes Hypothyroidism with Signs of Neoplastic Alterations. *PLoS ONE* **2012**, *7*, e29929. [CrossRef]
71. Frezzetti, D.; Reale, C.; Calì, G.; Nitsch, L.; Fagman, H.; Nilsson, O.; Scarfò, M.; De Vita, G.; Di Lauro, R. The microRNA-Processing Enzyme Dicer Is Essential for Thyroid Function. *PLoS ONE* **2011**, *6*, e27648. [CrossRef] [PubMed]
72. Schultz, K.A.P.; Williams, G.M.; Kamihara, J.; Stewart, D.R.; Harris, A.K.; Bauer, A.J.; Turner, J.; Shah, R.; Schneider, K.; Schneider, K.W.; et al. DICER1 and Associated Conditions: Identification of At-risk Individuals and Recommended Surveillance Strategies. *Clin. Cancer Res.* **2018**, *24*, 2251–2261. [CrossRef] [PubMed]
73. Rutter, M.M.; Jha, P.; Schultz, K.A.P.; Sheil, A.; Harris, A.K.; Bauer, A.J.; Field, A.L.; Geller, J.; Hill, D.A. DICER1Mutations and Differentiated Thyroid Carcinoma: Evidence of a Direct Association. *J. Clin. Endocrinol. Metab.* **2016**, *101*, 1–5. [CrossRef] [PubMed]
74. Cerami, E.; Gao, J.; Dogrusoz, U.; Gross, B.E.; Sumer, S.O.; Aksoy, B.A.; Jacobsen, A.; Byrne, C.J.; Heuer, M.L.; Larsson, E.; et al. The cBio Cancer Genomics Portal: An Open Platform for Exploring Multidimensional Cancer Genomics Data: Figure 1. *Cancer Discov.* **2012**, *2*, 401–404. [CrossRef] [PubMed]
75. Gao, J.; Aksoy, B.A.; Dogrusoz, U.; Dresdner, G.; Gross, B.; Sumer, S.O.; Sun, Y.; Jacobsen, A.; Sinha, R.; Larsson, E.; et al. Integrative Analysis of Complex Cancer Genomics and Clinical Profiles Using the cBioPortal. *Sci. Signal.* **2013**, *6*, pl1. [CrossRef]
76. cBioPortal for Cancer Genomics. Available online: https://www.cbioportal.org (accessed on 16 August 2020).
77. Cancer Genome Atlas Research Network. Integrated genomic characterization of papillary thyroid carcinoma. *Cell* **2014**, *159*, 676–690. [CrossRef]
78. Landa, I.; Ibrahimpasic, T.; Boucai, L.; Sinha, R.; Knauf, J.A.; Shah, R.H.; Dogan, S.; Ricarte-Filho, J.C.; Krishnamoorthy, G.P.; Xu, B.; et al. Genomic and transcriptomic hallmarks of poorly differentiated and anaplastic thyroid cancers. *J. Clin. Investig.* **2016**, *126*, 1052–1066. [CrossRef]
79. Chernock, R.D.; Rivera, B.; Borrelli, N.; Hill, D.A.; Fahiminiya, S.; Shah, T.; Chong, A.-S.; Aqil, B.; Mehrad, M.; Giordano, T.J.; et al. Poorly differentiated thyroid carcinoma of childhood and adolescence: A distinct entity characterized by DICER1 mutations. *Mod. Pathol.* **2020**, *33*, 1264–1274. [CrossRef]
80. Wasserman, J.D.; Sabbaghian, N.; Fahiminiya, S.; Chami, R.; Mete, O.; Acker, M.; Wu, M.K.; Shlien, A.; De Kock, L.; Foulkes, W.D. DICER1 Mutations Are Frequent in Adolescent-Onset Papillary Thyroid Carcinoma. *J. Clin. Endocrinol. Metab.* **2018**, *103*, 2009–2015. [CrossRef]
81. Canberk, S.; Ferreira, J.C.; Pereira, L.; Batısta, R.; Vieira, A.F.; Soares, P.; Simões, M.S.; Máximo, V. Analyzing the Role of DICER1 Germline Variations in Papillary Thyroid Carcinoma. *Eur. Thyroid J.* **2020**, 1–8. [CrossRef]

82. Rivera, B.; Nadaf, J.; Fahiminiya, S.; Apellaniz-Ruiz, M.; Saskin, A.; Chong, A.-S.; Sharma, S.; Wagener, R.; Revil, T.; Condello, V.; et al. DGCR8 microprocessor defect characterizes familial multinodular goiter with schwannomatosis. *J. Clin. Investig.* **2020**, *130*, 1479–1490. [CrossRef] [PubMed]
83. Kastenhuber, E.R.; Lowe, S.W. Putting p53 in Context. *Cell* **2017**, *170*, 1062–1078. [CrossRef] [PubMed]
84. Goldgar, D.E.; Easton, D.F.; Cannon-Albright, L.A.; Skolnick, M.H. Systematic Population-Based Assessment of Cancer Risk in First-Degree Relatives of Cancer Probands. *J. Natl. Cancer Inst.* **1994**, *86*, 1600–1608. [CrossRef] [PubMed]
85. Hemminki, K.; Eng, C.; Chen, B. Familial Risks for Nonmedullary Thyroid Cancer. *J. Clin. Endocrinol. Metab.* **2005**, *90*, 5747–5753. [CrossRef]
86. Bauer, A.J. Clinical Behavior and Genetics of Nonsyndromic, Familial Nonmedullary Thyroid Cancer. *Front. Horm. Res.* **2013**, *41*, 141–148. [CrossRef]
87. Capezzone, M.; Marchisotta, S.; Cantara, S.; Busonero, G.; Brilli, L.; Pazaitou-Panayiotou, K.; Carli, A.F.; Caruso, G.; Toti, P.; Capitani, S.; et al. Familial non-medullary thyroid carcinoma displays the features of clinical anticipation suggestive of a distinct biological entity. *Endocr. Relat. Cancer* **2008**, *15*, 1075–1081. [CrossRef]
88. He, H.; Bronisz, A.; Liyanarachchi, S.; Nagy, R.; Li, W.; Huang, Y.; Akagi, K.; Saji, M.; Kula, D.; Wojcicka, A.; et al. SRGAP1 Is a Candidate Gene for Papillary Thyroid Carcinoma Susceptibility. *J. Clin. Endocrinol. Metab.* **2013**, *98*, E973–E980. [CrossRef]
89. Suh, I.; Filetti, S.; Vriens, M.R.; Guerrero, M.A.; Tumino, S.; Wong, M.; Shen, W.T.; Kebebew, E.; Duh, Q.-Y.; Clark, O.H. Distinct loci on chromosome 1q21 and 6q22 predispose to familial nonmedullary thyroid cancer: A SNP array-based linkage analysis of 38 families. *Surgery* **2009**, *146*, 1073–1080. [CrossRef]
90. He, H.; Nagy, R.; Liyanarachchi, S.; Jiao, H.; Li, W.; Suster, S.; Kere, J.; De La Chapelle, A. A Susceptibility Locus for Papillary Thyroid Carcinoma on Chromosome 8q24. *Cancer Res.* **2009**, *69*, 625–631. [CrossRef]
91. He, H.; Li, W.; Wu, D.; Nagy, R.; Liyanarachchi, S.; Akagi, K.; Jendrzejewski, J.; Jiao, H.; Hoag, K.; Wen, B.; et al. Ultra-Rare Mutation in Long-Range Enhancer Predisposes to Thyroid Carcinoma with High Penetrance. *PLoS ONE* **2013**, *8*, e61920. [CrossRef]
92. Ngan, E.S.W.; Lang, B.H.H.; Liu, T.; Shum, C.K.Y.; So, M.-T.; Lau, D.K.C.; Leon, T.Y.Y.; Cherny, S.S.; Tsai, S.Y.; Lo, C.-Y.; et al. A Germline Mutation (A339V) in Thyroid Transcription Factor-1 (TITF-1/NKX2.1) in Patients with Multinodular Goiter and Papillary Thyroid Carcinoma. *J. Natl. Cancer Inst.* **2009**, *101*, 162–175. [CrossRef] [PubMed]
93. McKay, J.D.; Thompson, D.B.; Lesueur, F.; Stankov, K.; Pastore, A.; Watfah, C.; Strolz, S.; Riccabona, G.; Moncayo, R.C.; Romeo, G.; et al. Evidence for interaction between the TCO and NMTC1 loci in familial non-medullary thyroid cancer. *J. Med. Genet.* **2004**, *41*, 407–412. [CrossRef] [PubMed]
94. Medapati, M.R.; Dahlmann, M.; Ghavami, S.; Pathak, K.A.; Lucman, L.; Klonisch, T.; Hoang-Vu, C.; Stein, U.; Hombach-Klonisch, S. RAGE Mediates the Pro-Migratory Response of Extracellular S100A4 in Human Thyroid Cancer Cells. *Thyroid* **2015**, *25*, 514–527. [CrossRef] [PubMed]
95. Burgess, J.R.; Duffield, A.; Wilkinson, S.J.; Ware, R.; Greenaway, T.M.; Percival, J.; Hoffman, L. Two Families with an Autosomal Dominant Inheritance Pattern for Papillary Carcinoma of the Thyroid. *J. Clin. Endocrinol. Metab.* **1997**, *82*, 345–348. [CrossRef]
96. Bakhsh, A.; Kirov, G.; Gregory, J.W.; Williams, E.D.; Ludgate, M. A new form of familial multi-nodular goitre with progression to differentiated thyroid cancer. *Endocr.-Relat. Cancer* **2006**, *13*, 475–483. [CrossRef]
97. Franceschi, S.; Preston-Martin, S.; Maso, L.D.; Negri, E.; La Vecchia, C.; Mack, W.J.; McTiernan, A.; Kolonel, L.; Mark, S.D.; Mabuchi, K.; et al. A pooled analysis of case—Control studies of thyroid cancer. IV. Benign thyroid diseases. *Cancer Causes Control.* **1999**, *10*, 583–595. [CrossRef]
98. Gudmundsson, J.; Sulem, P.; Gudbjartsson, D.F.; Jonasson, J.G.; Sigurdsson, A.; Bergthorsson, J.T.; He, H.; Blondal, T.; Geller, F.; Jakobsdottir, M.; et al. Common variants on 9q22.33 and 14q13.3 predispose to thyroid cancer in European populations. *Nat. Genet.* **2009**, *41*, 460–464. [CrossRef]
99. Gudmundsson, J.; Sulem, P.; Gudbjartsson, D.F.; Jonasson, J.G.; Masson, G.; He, H.; Jonasdottir, A.; Sigurdsson, A.; Stacey, S.N.; Johannsdottir, H.; et al. Discovery of common variants associated with low TSH levels and thyroid cancer risk. *Nat. Genet.* **2012**, *44*, 319–322. [CrossRef]

100. Takahashi, M.; Saenko, V.A.; Rogounovitch, T.I.; Kawaguchi, T.; Drozd, V.M.; Takigawa-Imamura, H.; Akulevich, N.M.; Ratanajaraya, C.; Mitsutake, N.; Takamura, N.; et al. The FOXE1 locus is a major genetic determinant for radiation-related thyroid carcinoma in Chernobyl. *Hum. Mol. Genet.* **2010**, *19*, 2516–2523. [CrossRef]

101. Köhler, A.; Chen, B.; Gemignani, F.; Elisei, R.; Romei, C.; Figlioli, G.; Cipollini, M.; Cristaudo, A.; Bambi, F.; Hoffmann, P.; et al. Genome-Wide Association Study on Differentiated Thyroid Cancer. *J. Clin. Endocrinol. Metab.* **2013**, *98*, E1674–E1681. [CrossRef]

102. Son, H.-Y.; Hwangbo, Y.; Yoo, S.-K.; Im, S.-W.; Yang, S.D.; Kwak, S.-J.; Park, M.S.; Kwak, S.H.; Cho, S.W.; Ryu, J.S.; et al. Genome-wide association and expression quantitative trait loci studies identify multiple susceptibility loci for thyroid cancer. *Nat. Commun.* **2017**, *8*, 15966. [CrossRef] [PubMed]

103. Gudmundsson, J.; Thorleifsson, G.; Sigurdsson, J.K.; Stefansdottir, L.; Jonasson, J.G.; Gudjonsson, S.A.; Gudbjartsson, D.F.; Masson, G.; Johannsdottir, H.; Halldorsson, G.H.; et al. A genome-wide association study yields five novel thyroid cancer risk loci. *Nat. Commun.* **2017**, *8*, 14517. [CrossRef] [PubMed]

104. Nikitski, A.V.; Rogounovitch, T.I.; Bychkov, A.; Takahashi, M.; Yoshiura, K.-I.; Mitsutake, N.; Kawaguchi, T.; Matsuse, M.; Drozd, V.M.; Demidchik, Y.; et al. Genotype Analyses in the Japanese and Belarusian Populations Reveal Independent Effects of rs965513 and rs1867277 but Do Not Support the Role of FOXE1 Polyalanine Tract Length in Conferring Risk for Papillary Thyroid Carcinoma. *Thyroid* **2017**, *27*, 224–235. [CrossRef] [PubMed]

105. Landa, I.; Ruiz-Llorente, S.; Montero-Conde, C.; Inglada-Pérez, L.; Schiavi, F.; Leskelä, S.; Pita, G.; Milne, R.; Maravall, J.; Ramos, I.; et al. The Variant rs1867277 in FOXE1 Gene Confers Thyroid Cancer Susceptibility through the Recruitment of USF1/USF2 Transcription Factors. *PLoS Genet.* **2009**, *5*, e1000637. [CrossRef]

106. Nikitski, A.; Saenko, V.; Shimamura, M.; Nakashima, M.; Matsuse, M.; Suzuki, K.; Rogounovitch, T.I.; Bogdanova, T.; Shibusawa, N.; Yamada, M.; et al. Targeted Foxe1 Overexpression in Mouse Thyroid Causes the Development of Multinodular Goiter But Does Not Promote Carcinogenesis. *Endocrinology* **2016**, *157*, 2182–2195. [CrossRef]

107. Wang, Y.; He, H.; Li, W.; Phay, J.; Shen, R.; Yu, L.; Hancioglu, B.; De La Chapelle, A. MYH9 binds to lncRNA genePTCSC2and regulates FOXE1 in the 9q22 thyroid cancer risk locus. *Proc. Natl. Acad. Sci. USA* **2017**, *114*, 474–479. [CrossRef]

108. Jones, A.M.; Howarth, K.M.; Martin, L.; Gorman, M.; Mihai, R.; Moss, L.; Auton, A.; Lemon, C.; Mehanna, H.; Mohan, H.; et al. Thyroid cancer susceptibility polymorphisms: Confirmation of loci on chromosomes 9q22 and 14q13, validation of a recessive 8q24 locus and failure to replicate a locus on 5q24. *J. Med. Genet.* **2012**, *49*, 158–163. [CrossRef]

109. Jendrzejewski, J.; He, H.; Radomska, H.S.; Li, W.; Tomsic, J.; Liyanarachchi, S.; Davuluri, R.V.; Nagy, R.; De La Chapelle, A. The polymorphism rs944289 predisposes to papillary thyroid carcinoma through a large intergenic noncoding RNA gene of tumor suppressor type. *Proc. Natl. Acad. Sci. USA* **2012**, *109*, 8646–8651. [CrossRef]

110. Goedert, L.; Plaça, J.R.; Fuziwara, C.S.; Machado, M.C.R.; Plaça, D.R.; Almeida, P.P.; Sanches, T.P.; Dos Santos, J.F.; Corveloni, A.C.; Pereira, I.E.G.; et al. Identification of Long Noncoding RNAs Deregulated in Papillary Thyroid Cancer and Correlated with BRAFV600E Mutation by Bioinformatics Integrative Analysis. *Sci. Rep.* **2017**, *7*, 1662. [CrossRef]

111. Jendrzejewski, J.; Thomas, A.; Liyanarachchi, S.; Eiterman, A.; Tomsic, J.; He, H.; Radomska, H.S.; Li, W.; Nagy, R.; Sworczak, K.; et al. PTCSC3 Is Involved in Papillary Thyroid Carcinoma Development by Modulating S100A4 Gene Expression. *J. Clin. Endocrinol. Metab.* **2015**, *100*, E1370–E1377. [CrossRef]

112. Cantara, S.; Capuano, S.; Formichi, C.; Pisu, M.; Capezzone, M.; Pacini, F. Lack of germline A339V mutation in thyroid transcription factor-1 (TITF-1/NKX2.1) gene in familial papillary thyroid cancer. *Thyroid Res.* **2010**, *3*, 4. [CrossRef] [PubMed]

113. He, H.; Li, W.; Liyanarachchi, S.; Wang, Y.; Yu, L.; Genutis, L.K.; Maharry, S.; Phay, J.E.; Shen, R.; Brock, P.; et al. The Role of NRG1 in the Predisposition to Papillary Thyroid Carcinoma. *J. Clin. Endocrinol. Metab.* **2018**, *103*, 1369–1379. [CrossRef] [PubMed]

114. Coe, E.A.; Tan, J.Y.; Shapiro, M.; Louphrasitthiphol, P.; Bassett, A.R.; Marques, A.C.; Goding, C.R.; Vance, K.W. The MITF-SOX10 regulated long non-coding RNA DIRC3 is a melanoma tumour suppressor. *PLoS Genet.* **2019**, *15*, e1008501. [CrossRef] [PubMed]

115. Świerniak, M.; Wójcicka, A.; Czetwertyńska, M.; Długosińska, J.; Stachlewska, E.; Gierlikowski, W.; Kot, A.; Górnicka, B.; Koperski, Ł.; Bogdańska, M.; et al. Association between GWAS-Derived rs966423 Genetic Variant and Overall Mortality in Patients with Differentiated Thyroid Cancer. *Clin. Cancer Res.* **2016**, *22*, 1111–1119. [CrossRef]
116. Hińcza, K.; Kowalik, A.; Pałyga, I.; Walczyk, A.; Gąsior-Perczak, D.; Mikina, E.; Trybek, T.; Szymonek, M.; Gadawska-Juszczyk, K.; Zajkowska, K.; et al. Does the TT Variant of the rs966423 Polymorphism in DIRC3 Affect the Stage and Clinical Course of Papillary Thyroid Cancer? *Cancers* **2020**, *12*, 423. [CrossRef]
117. Liyanarachchi, S.; Gudmundsson, J.; Ferkingstad, E.; He, H.; Jonasson, J.G.; Tragante, V.; Asselbergs, F.W.; Xu, L.; Kiemeney, L.A.; Netea-Maier, R.T.; et al. Assessing thyroid cancer risk using polygenic risk scores. *Proc. Natl. Acad. Sci. USA* **2020**, *117*, 5997–6002. [CrossRef]
118. Capezzone, M.; Cantara, S.; Marchisotta, S.; Filetti, S.; De Santi, M.M.; Rossi, B.; Ronga, G.; Durante, C.; Pacini, F. Short Telomeres, Telomerase Reverse Transcriptase Gene Amplification, and Increased Telomerase Activity in the Blood of Familial Papillary Thyroid Cancer Patients. *J. Clin. Endocrinol. Metab.* **2008**, *93*, 3950–3957. [CrossRef]
119. He, M.; Bian, B.; Gesuwan, K.; Gulati, N.; Zhang, L.; Nilubol, N.; Kebebew, E. Telomere Length Is Shorter in Affected Members of Families with Familial Nonmedullary Thyroid Cancer. *Thyroid* **2013**, *23*, 301–307. [CrossRef]
120. Cantara, S.; Capuano, S.; Capezzone, M.; Benigni, M.; Pisu, M.; Marchisotta, S.; Pacini, F. Lack of Mutations of the Telomerase RNA Component in Familial Papillary Thyroid Cancer with Short Telomeres. *Thyroid* **2012**, *22*, 363–368. [CrossRef]
121. He, H.; Li, W.; Comiskey, D.F.; Liyanarachchi, S.; Nieminen, T.T.; Wang, Y.; DeLap, K.E.; Brock, P.; De La Chapelle, A. A Truncating Germline Mutation of TINF2 in Individuals with Thyroid Cancer or Melanoma Results in Longer Telomeres. *Thyroid* **2020**, *30*, 204–213. [CrossRef]
122. Srivastava, A.; Miao, B.; Skopelitou, D.; Kumar, V.; Kumar, A.; Paramasivam, N.; Bonora, E.; Hemminki, K.; Foersti, A.; Bandapalli, O.R. A Germline Mutation in the POT1 Gene Is a Candidate for Familial Non-Medullary Thyroid Cancer. *Cancers* **2020**, *12*, 1441. [CrossRef] [PubMed]
123. Wilson, T.L.-S.; Hattangady, N.; Lerario, A.M.; Williams, C.; Koeppe, E.; Quinonez, S.; Osborne, J.; Cha, K.B.; Else, T. A new POT1 germline mutation—expanding the spectrum of POT1-associated cancers. *Fam. Cancer* **2017**, *16*, 561–566. [CrossRef] [PubMed]
124. Richard, M.A.; Lupo, P.J.; Morton, L.M.; Yasui, Y.A.; Sapkota, Y.A.; Arnold, M.A.; Aubert, G.; Neglia, J.P.; Turcotte, L.M.; Leisenring, W.M.; et al. Genetic variation in POT1 and risk of thyroid subsequent malignant neoplasm: A report from the Childhood Cancer Survivor Study. *PLoS ONE* **2020**, *15*, e0228887. [CrossRef] [PubMed]
125. Tomsic, J.; Fultz, R.; Liyanarachchi, S.; Genutis, L.K.; Wang, Y.; Li, W.; Volinia, S.; Jazdzewski, K.; He, H.; Wakely, P.E., Jr.; et al. Variants in microRNA genes in familial papillary thyroid carcinoma. *Oncotarget* **2017**, *8*, 6475–6482. [CrossRef]
126. Tomsic, J.; He, H.; Akagi, K.; Liyanarachchi, S.; Pan, Q.; Bertani, B.; Nagy, R.; Symer, D.E.; Blencowe, B.J.; De La Chapelle, A. A germline mutation in SRRM2, a splicing factor gene, is implicated in papillary thyroid carcinoma predisposition. *Sci. Rep.* **2015**, *5*, 10566. [CrossRef]
127. Orois, A.; Gara, S.K.; Mora, M.; Halperin, I.; Martínez, S.; Alfayate, R.; Kebebew, E.; Oriola, J. NOP53 as A Candidate Modifier Locus for Familial Non-Medullary Thyroid Cancer. *Genes* **2019**, *10*, 899. [CrossRef]
128. Gara, S.K.; Jia, L.; Merino, M.J.; Agarwal, S.K.; Zhang, L.; Cam, M.; Patel, D.; Kebebew, E. Germline HABP2 Mutation Causing Familial Nonmedullary Thyroid Cancer. *N. Engl. J. Med.* **2015**, *373*, 448–455. [CrossRef]
129. Tomsic, J.; He, H.; de la Chapelle, A. HABP2 Mutation and Nonmedullary Thyroid Cancer. *N. Engl. J. Med.* **2015**, *373*, 2086. [CrossRef]
130. Tomsic, J.; Fultz, R.; Liyanarachchi, S.; He, H.; Senter, L.; De La Chapelle, A. HABP2 G534E Variant in Papillary Thyroid Carcinoma. *PLoS ONE* **2016**, *11*, e0146315. [CrossRef]
131. Kowalik, A.; Gąsior-Perczak, D.; Gromek, M.; Siołek, M.; Walczyk, A.; Pałyga, I.; Chłopek, M.; Kopczyński, J.; Mężyk, R.; Kowalska, A.; et al. The p.G534E variant of HABP2 is not associated with sporadic papillary thyroid carcinoma in a Polish population. *Oncotarget* **2017**, *8*, 58304–58308. [CrossRef]
132. Zhu, J.; Wu, K.; Lin, Z.; Bai, S.; Wu, J.; Li, P.; Xue, H.; Du, J.; Shen, B.; Wang, H.; et al. Identification of susceptibility gene mutations associated with the pathogenesis of familial nonmedullary thyroid cancer. *Mol. Genet. Genom. Med.* **2019**, *7*, e1015. [CrossRef] [PubMed]

133. Sarquis, M.; Moraes, D.C.; Bastos-Rodrigues, L.; Azevedo, P.G.; Ramos, A.V.; Reis, F.V.; Dande, P.V.; Paim, I.; Friedman, E.; De Marco, L. Germline Mutations in Familial Papillary Thyroid Cancer. *Endocr. Pathol.* **2020**, *31*, 14–20. [CrossRef] [PubMed]
134. Siołek, M.; Cybulski, C.; Gąsior-Perczak, D.; Kowalik, A.; Kozak-Klonowska, B.; Kowalska, A.; Chłopek, M.; Kluźniak, W.; Wokołorczyk, D.; Pałyga, I.; et al. CHEK2 mutations and the risk of papillary thyroid cancer. *Int. J. Cancer* **2015**, *137*, 548–552. [CrossRef] [PubMed]

Publisher's Note: MDPI stays neutral with regard to jurisdictional claims in published maps and institutional affiliations.

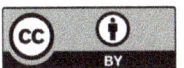

© 2020 by the authors. Licensee MDPI, Basel, Switzerland. This article is an open access article distributed under the terms and conditions of the Creative Commons Attribution (CC BY) license (http://creativecommons.org/licenses/by/4.0/).

MDPI
St. Alban-Anlage 66
4052 Basel
Switzerland
Tel. +41 61 683 77 34
Fax +41 61 302 89 18
www.mdpi.com

Genes Editorial Office
E-mail: genes@mdpi.com
www.mdpi.com/journal/genes

www.ingramcontent.com/pod-product-compliance
Lightning Source LLC
LaVergne TN
LVHW070043120526
838202LV00101B/421